Social Skills and Autistic Spectrum Disorders

Social Skills and Autistic Spectrum Disorders

Lynn Plimley and
Maggie Bowen

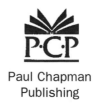

Paul Chapman
Publishing

Paul Chapman Publishing
A SAGE Publications Company
1 Oliver's Yard
55 City Road
London EC1Y 1SP

SAGE Publications Inc
2455 Teller Road
Thousand Oaks, California 91320

SAGE Publications India Pvt Ltd
B 1/I 1 Mohan Cooperative Industrial Area
Mathura Road, Post Bag 7
New Delhi 110 044

Library of Congress Control Number 2006932496

A catalogue record for this book is available from the
British Library

ISBN-1-4129-2312-3   ISBN-978-1-4129-2312-5
ISBN-1-4129-2313-1   ISBN-978-1-4129-2313-2 (pbk)

Typeset by C&M Digitals (P) Ltd., Chennai, India
Printed in Great Britain by Cromwell Press Ltd, Trowbridge, Wiltshire
Printed on paper from sustainable resources

Contents

Acknowledgements

Our sincere thanks go to a range of people who have helped us gather evidence for this book, namely colleagues on the Webautism Team (**www.webautism.bham.ac.uk**), SNAP Cymru, Enid Moore, Denise Hawkins and Jonathan Morgan and young people with ASD in North Wales, Jude Bowen and NoMAD. We would like to thank PAPA, Northern Ireland for their inspiring approaches to individuals with ASD and their families.

The authors wish to acknowledge the collaborative contribution of Andrea Macleod, Lecturer in ASD, School of Education, University of Birmingham to Chapters 2, 3, 5 & 7. Her knowledge and experience of issues affecting the population of adults with ASD adds an important dimension.

Lynn Plimley

Lynn Plimley trained to teach children with special educational needs in the mid-70s, and has worked with children with ASD since 1979.

She has worked in generic special schools for primary-aged children and in residential schools for those with SLD. She also spent a year in a multi-disciplinary team to support the inclusion of children with learning difficulties in mainstream schools.

After spending three years as a Deputy Head in a large special school, she joined a local autistic society and for three years developed their training and educational information services, going on to become the first Principal of Coddington Court School for children aged 8–19 with ASD in Herefordshire.

She has also worked indirectly with adults and young people on the autistic spectrum.

Currently she works part-time as a Lecturer in ASD at Birmingham University with their web-based course (www.webautism.bham.ac.uk). She also works for Autism Cymru building up a series 3 National Fora for mainstream secondary school teachers, primary school teachers and special school teachers, to share good practice, and co-deliver LEA training with Maggie Bowen.

She has also worked in a consultancy role for Prior's Court School in Berkshire with teaching and care staff.

She tutors M.Ed dissertation students for the Course in ASD (Distance Learning) and is a member of the internationally respected Autism team, based at the University of Birmingham's School of Education, led by Professor Rita Jordan.

The Autism team has recently undertaken commissioned work to Develop an ASD information website and fact sheets for Primary Care Practitioners for NES–NHS in Scotland and a review of services for young people with Asperger syndrome in Northern Ireland, for the Northern Ireland Commissioner for Children and Young People (NICCY).

She is the book editor and an Editorial Board member of the *Good Autism Practice, Journal*. Lynn has built up a national profile of training in the importance of understanding the condition of autistic spectrum disorders for schools and care establishments.

Maggie Bowen

Maggie gained her academic and professional qualifications at universities in Aberystwyth, Leeds and Bangor. She began her teaching career in a school for children with severe learning difficulties (SLD), and went on to work as a Community Liaison Teacher for individuals with SLD. She has been a Team Inspector of secondary and special schools, and a Threshold Assessor, and has worked as part of a multi-agency team and been responsible for developing a range of new services for individuals of all ages with a SLD.

She was Programme Leader for Special Educational Needs courses and the MA in Education at the North East Wales Institute of Higher Education (NEWI). In 2000, she worked as consultant/writer for the ACCAC (Wales) document *A Structure for Success. Guidance on National Curriculum and Autistic Spectrum Disorders'*. She has worked for the Welsh Assembly Government (WAG) as Development officer for inclusion in Wales with a specific responsibility for Autistic Spectrum Disorders (ASDs), Able and Talented and SEN Training. She continues to work closely with the WAG on ASD matters.

She joined the team at Autism Cymru as Head of Public and Voluntary Sector Partnerships/Deputy CEO in January 2005. She has published on a range of SEN issues in books and journals, and is still committed to training and consultancy work with a range of practitioners from health, social services, education, the criminal justice system and the emergency services. She is a Registered Practitioner with the Higher Education Academy.

How to use this book

This book is one in the series entitled 'The Autistic Spectrum Disorders Toolkit'. It focuses on the variety of social skills issues that a person with autistic spectrum disorders (ASD) may face, whatever their age or level of functioning. Autism Cymru host a forum for teachers and workers in primary secondary and special schools, where there is an opportunity to share best practice and also their concerns about the young people in their care. The content of this book refers to some of the discussions that have taken place at these meetings and has therefore been shaped by the work of experienced practitioners.

Throughout the book, readers are asked to examine issues from the perspective of the individual with ASD rather than to adopt a traditional behavioural approach to the situation. Case studies of best practice and strategies suggested are designed to be of practical help to the reader. Readers are also given the opportunity to reflect on their own practice and enhance their professional development by using the 'Reflective Oasis' contained in each chapter.

The impact of the triad of impairments on social skills development

This chapter will give a brief description of the term Autistic Spectrum Disorders (ASD). It will discuss the difficulties that may arise in social skills development, based on the triad of impairment. It is an introductory chapter that sets the scene for the rest of the book.

ASD: a historical overview

The condition of autistic spectrum disorders is one that has had an array of other names (most with the term 'autism' mentioned somewhere) throughout its relatively short diagnostic lifespan. The conditions of autism and also of Asperger syndrome were described in the mid-1940s by two separate Austrian medical practitioners: Leo Kanner, a child psychiatrist, and Hans Asperger, a paediatrician. This does not mean, however, that the condition has existed only since that time. It is possible that autism or its characteristics have existed through time (Frith, 1989; Waltz, 2005).

Currently, we recognise the work of both Kanner, who described a set of characteristics, also termed 'Kanner's autism', classic autism (1943), and that of Asperger, who described similar characteristics and some physical differences. These two contemporaries published their research at around the same time, but by advantage of living in the USA, Kanner's work became known to the English-speaking population a long time before Asperger's, who published in Austria in German (1944), compared with an English account of Asperger's work by Wing (1981). A fuller historical picture can be gained from reading Wing (1996), Frith (1989) and Jordan (1999).

The triad of impairments

The current terminology is 'autistic (or autism) spectrum disorder/s' (Wing, 1996). To have a basic understanding of the condition, it is important to know about the triad of impairments (Wing, 1988) – the three main areas of development where people on the autistic spectrum manifest differences – which we outline in the following paragraphs.

Social interaction

- Preference for individual activities
- Apparent aloofness
- Indifference towards others
- More adult-oriented than peer-oriented
- Likely to exhibit different spontaneous responses
- Passive acceptance of contact
- Lack of empathy
- Failure to appreciate significant others
- Poor understanding of social rules and conventions
- Unable to seek comfort at times of distress.

Wing and Gould (1979) believe that there is also a sub-group of three distinct character/behaviour types in social interaction.

Aloof

This refers to the most commonly manifest characteristics and describes those people with ASD who behave as if you are not there, do not respond to your interactions, and lead you to the place/activity that they want rather than requesting it.

Passive

This may be the least common sub-group who are completely passive in their interactions with others; they will accept interaction and become a willing 'participant' in whatever is happening.

Active but odd

These characteristics are evident in those who wish to have social contact but lack a means of initiating it in a socially appropriate way. So they may hold a gaze too long, sit too close or respond in an unpredictable way.

Communication

- Little desire to communicate socially
- Lack of understanding non-verbal gestures of others
- Not appreciative of need to communicate information
- Idiosyncratic use of words and phrases
- Prescribed content of speech
- May talk at, rather than to
- Poor grasp of abstract concepts and feelings
- Literal understanding of words and phrases
- Does not 'get' subtle jokes
- Will develop expression before understanding.

Rigidity of behaviour and thought

- May have stereotyped play activities
- Can become attached to repetition of movement or certain objects or routines
- Complex order of play/activity
- Cannot deviate from one way of doing things
- May be tolerant of situations and then overreact to something minor
- May develop rituals that have to be completed
- Can have extreme physical rituals – e.g. spinning, rocking
- Can develop extreme behaviours to avoid certain stimuli.

Areas of difference in the child's development have to be noted by the age of 3 years. This is not to say that diagnosis happens only in early childhood, but by reviewing early developmental milestones, a diagnostician will ask questions of parents/carers about the child's levels of communication and play before the age of 3.

The recognised descriptors for diagnosis are contained in two separate medical reference books: the *ICD 10 – International Classification of Diseases Version 10* (1993), which is compiled by the World Health Organisation, and the *Diagnostic and Statistical Manual of Mental Health version IV* (1994), which is compiled by the American Psychiatric Association.

Learning from individuals with ASD

A number of individuals with ASD now write and talk about their particular way of thinking and how this impacts on their social interaction and communication. It is useful at this point to pause and consider some quotations before exploring issues in greater detail. It is often very important to try to see things from the perspective of the individual with ASD when considering strategies that might help.

> Asperger's Syndrome subdues my ability to think straight and rationally, to keep calm and collected even in the most trivial of circumstances. I'm not trying to blame what could be a character flaw on my condition, but that a significant number of my Asperger friends claim to experience a similar reduced capacity for calm and rational thought in the face of adversity. (Nita Jackson, 2002, p. 66)

> I think of it like this: society is one big mirror consisting of billions of individual mirrors, one carried by each individual, the majority of which reflect each other. Asperger people have frosted mirrors, so the reflections they receive are clouded and undefined. Some mirrors eventually clear, gaining the Asperger person a legible, possibly even nearly mainstream, understanding of reality. Some verge on the slightly blurred, some make it to the half way sign, others fall marginally below, and others never change. (Nita Jackson, 2002, p. 68)

> People probably assume I am stuck up and rude because of inappropriate responses. For example I did not know I was supposed to say hi to people when they said hi to me until I was 13 and I was not able to make it a habit until the age of 14. It is still difficult to understand some things. Like if someone gives you something (like someone passes you a piece of paper) it is appropriate to say thank you. I have trouble determining exactly which situations to say thank you in, or how to say it, or reacting fast enough. (Quinn in Sainsbury, 2000, p. 78)

> Having fashion sense, keeping up with hygiene and socializing in larger groups of people were skills that only began to solidify for me in my years after graduating from high school. (Karen in Sainsbury, 2000, p. 81)

> Wishing to join a conversation or group activity … [people with Asperger's] will be completely unaware of the subtle ways of initiating contact 'appropriately', and will instead either blunder in an interrupting way, or hover around on the fringes of the group without awareness that their presence is seen as either ridiculous or creepy or even threatening. (Joseph in Sainsbury, 2000, p. 83)

> I am always being told off for standing too close to people and following them around all the time but it is difficult to know when it is right to follow

someone around and carry on talking and when the conversation has ended and I am to leave them alone. I will never be able to tell if someone is bored unless they tell me, and even then I have to admit that I sometimes carry on talking if it is about my favourite topic. It is easy to know things in theory but not so easy to carry them out. (Luke Jackson, 2002, p. 164)

Autistics can be devastated and not cry. They can react wildly to events others treat as trivial. They can and do miss loved ones who have died. They can be deeply scarred for years following the loss of someone they feel attached to. Not only have they lost someone that they enjoyed being around, their routine has altered, as well, so they feel afraid. (Jasmine Lee-O'Neil, 1999, p. 81)

REFLECTIVE OASIS

Consider the quotations you have just read.

Have any of them helped you to understand a person with ASD that you know a little better?

The impact of the triad of impairments on social skills development

Difficulties in social communication

As we form relationships with families, friends and others, there is a number of things we take for granted. We learn to detect mood and appreciate that using a particular tone of voice has an implied meaning. For individuals with ASD, this can be a complicated process. Luke Jackson (2002) says how difficult it can sometimes be to understand what is required when an emphasis on just one word in a sentence can alter its meaning quite dramatically. Here is his example:

I can't do that – implies I can't but maybe someone else can.

I **can't** do that – implies it is not possible.

I can't do **that** – implies I can't do that, but may be able to do something else.

Our mood is often reflected in our body language – for example, arms folded, head down can show that we are unhappy even if the words we speak state that we are not. We know when people are getting bored with our conversation because their body language can show us this. If we are bored listening to someone with ASD talking about a topic of particular interest, loss of eye contact, huffing, puffing and moving away will not end the conversation!

Idioms are used regularly by us in everyday language, e.g. 'It's raining cats and dogs', 'On cloud nine' and 'Pigs might fly'. Phrases such as these can be confusing to individuals with ASD who take things very literally. The language of the classroom can also cause confusion. Consider just a few of the phrases we hear in school:

'Red table go to the Hall'

'Make a circle'

'Line up'

'Go and wash your hands in the toilet'

'Look at the board and I will go through it with you'.

The social demands of others can often cause anxiety. It is common for us to make polite conversation about the weather, but for some individuals with ASD this would be a pointless exercise. They would have to put a great deal of effort into an activity which they considered to be of no value. We can see what the weather is like, so why speak about it?

Any conversation with an individual with ASD will need to be specific and unambiguous. We often use polite language implying that there is a choice when actually there is not, e.g. saying 'Shall we go to Assembly?' implies a choice when really we are saying, 'We will go to Assembly now'. If using instructions, it is important to name the individual even if the instruction is aimed at a group. Jackson (2002) says that maybe it is a good idea to have practice times to show the person with ASD exaggerated signs of when it is OK to talk and when it is time to listen.

Difficulties in social relationships

The first-person quotations above show that it can be difficult to join groups and make friends. Sometimes this leads to feelings of isolation and even depression. Strategies how to make and maintain friendships may need to be learned, especially as, on the surface, some individuals (like Quinn, quoted previously) can be considered insensitive or egocentric. Although we say honesty is the best policy, we know that sometimes we need to tell 'little white lies' to keep our friends and family happy. For example, if we think a girl friend looks as if she has put on weight, we will avoid telling her. Individuals with ASD can be very honest – they like to tell it as it is and can often cause offence without being aware of doing so. They can also find it very difficult to understand how to react to other people's feelings and can respond in an inappropriate way in a sensitive situation, e.g. a funeral. Sometimes their inappropriate behaviour in a public place can get them into serious trouble (see Chapter 6).

Rigidity of thought

Special interests

Many individuals with ASD have a 'special interest'. This can involve the love of a sport such as ice-skating, trampolining or judo or an interest in a particular topic such as trains, or a hobby such as stamp collecting. Often the special interest can be all-absorbing for the individual with ASD. This might be fine when they are in the company of people with the same interest or on their own, but can cause social difficulties when they are with people who do not share that interest. Children in particular will lose patience, and friendships will not be maintained. Special interests are of great value and importance to individuals with ASD; they can help relieve the stresses and strains of everyday life but must be used in a positive and flexible way in order to do this.

Insistence on rules and routines

People with ASD like structure in their lives and respond very well to rules and routines. They find it very difficult to cope with sudden changes in their daily routine. Nita Jackson (2002, p. 52) explains:

> I was sensitive to change. I was terrified of it, because change leapt into the unknown and I could not get my head around the concept of exactly what the unknown was. I was so sensitive to the ever changing world around me, and everything I did at school was dictated by others, so I had no control. To compensate I had to exert my control by building a definite routine out of school life.

Transfer of skills

Skills learnt in one situation are not automatically transferred or generalised to another similar situation. For example, if a person with ASD is taught to wash up at school, he/she will not easily be able to transfer these skills to the home. Something as simple as a different colour or shape of bowl, or a different brand of washing-up liquid in each place could cause confusion. This transfer of skills can also apply to social interaction as Darius (Sainsbury, 2000, p. 82) explains:

> I only recognize people if I see them in the same context and they wear the same clothes. It takes many years before I learn to recognize people in more than one situation or with different clothes. Even then meeting them in an unexpected situation/place will result in blank stares from me because I don't recognize them.

REFLECTIVE OASIS

Think of someone you know with ASD.

Do they have a circle of friends?

Do they belong to any clubs or social groups?

Have they ever encountered any difficulties in social situations?

If so, what did you do to help?

Points to remember

- The triad of impairments has an impact on the social skills development of individuals with ASD. It results in difficulties in social interaction, social communication and flexible thinking.
- People with ASD:
  - will experience difficulties in their interpretation of language and body signals, and this can lead to misunderstandings
  - often find it hard to make and maintain friends
  - like structure in their lives; they do not like change
  - cannot easily transfer skills from one situation to another.

2

Ages and stages – an overview of what issues might be encountered at different stages in the life cycle

The key defining features of the triad of impairments (Wing, 1988) present in everyone with a diagnosis of ASD, will have a marked impact in all areas of social skills, at all stages in life. Some of these features may help to alert the individual or their parent/carer to a difference in their development. Crucial differences in the way they communicate, follow their own pursuits or need to have a pattern of sameness and familiarity, are directly attributed to the triad's significant differences in social inter-action, communication and rigidity of thought and behaviour. By look-ing at some of the typical differences at stages through life, we will track how the impact of the triad and the interplay of its features may conspire to make a crucial difference in the experiences and development of a person.

Early infanthood

ASD is a pervasive developmental disorder rather than a congenital condition (one that someone is born with). As the person develops, the characteristics of ASD emerge. As a consequence, the majority of parents will say that there were particular times within the early part of their child's life when their development veered away from what they were expecting. Parents who have older children may know earlier that the child has a different pattern of development because they have had other children to compare with. For first-time parents, it may take longer to notice.

Some of the 'suspicious behaviours' which can alert the parent to developmental difference are:

- Desire for sameness
- Poor interactional skills: lack of recognition of significant others (mother, father, siblings, other children) and/or lack of wanting the attention of others in play, e.g. not holding up toys for approval or dropping toys for retrieval by others
- Slow development of a communication system – language is not developing or has developed in an unusual way – words are not used to convey meaning to others
- Language development that has slowed or stopped
- Not 'hearing' what others are saying – paying little attention to the communication of others
- Limited communication skills – lack of joint attention – not pointing out; not making vocalisations for others to copy and make into a game
- Liking for solitary and stereotyped play – playing with mechanical objects in a rote fashion (not varying play activity)
- Lining, selecting or sorting to a predictable pattern
- Preference for same activity and a liking for the familiar – indications of distress if routines are changed or situations or environments are new for them
- Not good at sharing or taking turns
- Prone to sensory overload.

A fuller outline of developmental differences in the early years features in ASD is given in Plimley, Bowen and Morgan (2007).

If we focus on the lack of interest in others and lack of appreciation of the significance of key people (parents, siblings, wider family members) in their lives, it summons our empathy for understanding what it may feel like to have a child who does not 'notice' you. It may lead to care-givers spending less and less time with the young infant, especially if they are not getting any feedback. Observation of typically developing children aged around 12 months will reveal a repertoire of behaviours that they have developed for getting the attention of others – pointing, crying, vocalising, vocalising louder, near-word utterances, sighs and funny noises and dropping objects intentionally. The infant with ASD may not employ any of these and may appear completely passive and unengaged. Ros Blackburn, an adult with autism, says her parents received a diagnosis of autism when she was around the age of 1, but she pays tribute to their persistence in not letting her 'get away with things' and keeping her at the heart of their family.

School age

Pre-school

As the child nears the age for starting school, they may have a placement in a nursery or pre-school playgroup. Both of these provisions are intended to broaden the skills and interests of the child, begin learning experiences as well as building up concentration and attention spans. They are also great places for socialisation with others of their age.

Many children, for a range of reasons, find going to a pre-school placement difficult. Parents and carers find it a difficult time too, as it marks the beginning of the separation between home and school. For many children with ASD it can represent a very confusing world. They may respond with anxiety and fear.

Consider the pre-school picture:

- Lots of other children in one place
- Not always the same children every day
- A highly stimulating environment – pictures, mobiles, models, as well as noise and music
- Strange adults, not always the same every day
- Lots of change of activity
- Free choice
- The pressure to join in with others
- The pressure to conform socially
- Group management.

Many provisions at this age and level concentrate on the enrichment of experience in a highly stimulating programme of events. At times, this may appear loud and chaotic.

The characterising features of ASD may mean this type of placement can be fraught with problems. Pre-school placements have an advantage that they are child-centred and they will see a variety of developmental delays and the manifestation of other disorders, which can help them provide for children who are different. They will also have good links to other pre-school services and a clear route for referral of children who need specialist intervention.

Recent research looking at predictors of school successes (Reed, Osborne and Waddington, 2006) looked at types of early teaching interventions, comparing a special nursery provision, a Portage delivered service and home-based applied behaviour analysis (ABA or sometimes called Lovaas – **www. lovaas.com**; Lovaas, 1987). For long-term outcomes, the authors make tentative conclusions that children with ASD who have taken part in ABA exhibit fewer behavioural problems when they go to school, but are less socialised than those who had been to special nursery. This could be directly attributable to the paramount role that adults have played in the ABA programme.

Apart from the interactional, communication and play differences that a child with ASD may show at this age, there can be developmental sticking points for the pre-school child with ASD. These are often feeding, toileting and sleeping. Parents may be grateful for extra input from the pre-school staff.

Transitions

Once the child is able to move on from their pre-school provision, staff and parents may find that the transition to a new setting will cause a regression to fears, behaviours and anxieties that had been worked through. The concept of a new setting with different routines, expectations and people will be something that many children with ASD will find difficult. Their preferences for the usual routines represent a security and consistency that they have depended upon. Parents and the existing provision need to plan and prepare for any changes in setting, preferably with the receiving school too, and this will be true at pre-school to primary school and every new change onwards. Repeated visits to a new school, introduction to new staff, photographs or videos of the new setting, having a 'buddy' who will guide and advise the child with ASD are some ways to make transitions easier. The more preparation that goes into moving to the new placement, the better. The child with ASD will need much more preparation than a sole visit and meeting a teacher once. This is something that parents and provisions can work on together.

As the child with ASD matures, the more obvious their social differences may become. Unlike most of their peers, they do not have a natural curiosity about others and will not divert their attention away from what they are doing to join socially with others. This will often be true in play routines, with the child with ASD opting to pace the perimeter of the playground, rather than join in games with peers. It is also evident in their speaking and listening skills. Children with ASD who have a good command of language will sometimes use it to monopolise the attention of others; focusing on conveying information about their own special interests is common. The role of the listener in this situation is to do just that – listen – and the individual with ASD may not be interested in what they have to offer. This may cause difficulties in primary classrooms where children are expected to exchange 'news', or in later schooling when pupils are expected to present information for a variety of different audiences. People with ASD report that they have difficulty recognising the ebb and flow of conversation (Grandin and Scariano, 1986) and cannot gauge where to butt in or when to leave pauses long enough for others to contribute. A visual clue, more obvious than an exchange of glances, may be needed to show where a person with ASD may contribute in a conversation.

This will also extend to their understanding of how to take turns – a critical feature of many school activities, especially where group tasks are concerned. The child with ASD may not have recognised the pattern of whose turn it is, particularly if the turn-taking relies on a social understanding of the situation. Giving a concrete object, something that can pass from hand to hand according to whose turn it is, or a paper dial to turn towards the person who takes the next turn, helps them understand the process. The more simple the symbol, the more portable it will be to take to places such as the playground, the PE hall or on a visit to the shops. There are many other school and home situations where turn-taking can also be practised, such as, whose turn to:

- do the washing up
- clean out the pet hamster
- sharpen the class pencils
- be first in the line (often a sticking point for children at schools)
- choose a DVD to watch
- lay the table.

Understanding turn-taking can be an important social skill for people with ASD to acquire because many social rules and expectations are reliant upon that understanding. Turn-taking will help a person with ASD to:

- be part of an orderly queue in the post office, petrol station, supermarket
- take a share in chores around the house
- allow others to pursue their preferred pastimes

- have a measured conversation with others
- give way to other vehicles
- open the door for others
- submerge their desire to have everything their way.

Turn-taking is an indication of our consideration for others and although the person with ASD may have to work hard at having that kind of empathy, being able to allow others their turn will be a visible indicator that they can allow others to have their needs satisfied too.

Other school considerations

Children with ASD in mainstream schools often respond well to having clear school rules and expectations. Once rules have been understood, the child with ASD may apply them rigidly and become the strongest advocate of justice for all. This may not win them many friends, especially as older childrens' misdemeanours may be increasingly subtle and daring. Children with ASD can be helped to understand the anomalies of social relationships – when to tell and when to keep quiet – via social stories (Gray, 1994; fuller explanation appears in Chapter 3), but essentially their naivety and wish to tell the truth should be applauded and used to their advantage. Where exploitation becomes a danger to their school experience – when others deliberately abuse their trust and naivety – more formal intervention by adults may be needed to protect the individual.

Schools and staff may have to put a great deal of effort into creating relationships for the pupil with ASD. They can often prefer solitary activity and sometimes their esoteric interests may mark them apart from their peers. Having a self-selected 'buddy' who will take an interest and offer friendship to the child may need to be artificially engineered initially before a mutual understanding develops; where this does not happen, devices such as 'circles of friends' (Whitaker et al., 1998; fuller explanation appears in Chapter 5) can effectively offer a selection of supporters for the child that follows them through an entire school phase. If this is not an option or does not succeed, then sometimes a close member of staff (teacher, support worker, lunchtime supervisor) can offer social support. This member of staff will need to become a 'champion' of the child with ASD to support their reputation in school, and work to build up a picture of social value to other school staff and pupils (a fuller explanation of this appears in Plimley and Bowen (2006a).

Secondary school

As children move into secondary schooling, elements of their core differences may be thrown into a sharper focus. While mainstream secondary schools carry an inbuilt structure of timetables, rooms, facilities and subject-specific teachers, the onus on the pupils is for increased independence and self-direction with a stronger group identity. The combination can be bewildering to children with ASD, and that is without the impending onset of puberty. Many secondary schools hold a strong focus on the group, rather than individuals, since their numbers of children are large and their approach cannot be as child-centred as primary school. Children may have a group membership of:

- a class or form
- a house system for sport and other activities
- a stream or ability banding for core subjects
- a team for some PE activities
- maybe gender-specific pursuits – PE, some vocational subjects.

These separate groups may bring a child into contact with a completely different set of peers or older children each time. For the child with ASD who finds many social interactions stressful, the expectations to form and perform as part of a group may be too much and lead to disaffection or outbursts of inappropriate behaviour. Both of these will mark out the child as being different from their peers and the latter may bring the attention of more formal school sanctions.

The social mores of attending a mainstream secondary school require children to implicitly follow the rules of the school, but also the unwritten rules of being a growing teenager. The pressure on children almost as soon as they move into secondary school is to conform to the norm of their peer group and not to 'make waves'. Those permitted a more individual identity within their peer group are either the class entertainers (for light relief) or the class toughies (whom most have a fear of). The child who ignores or misunderstands these unwritten social rules can be the subject of social isolation or, in more extreme cases, bullying. Secondary school therefore can represent a social minefield for a child with ASD.

The curricular demands of the later stages of primary and into secondary education may also be a pressure upon the child with ASD. As a child progresses through their schooling, the subject distinction becomes sharper. The way in which the pupil is expected to interact with subject-content moves away from prescriptive tasks to practise skills and concepts, to more synthesis of ideas and generalisation of what has been learnt. The child with ASD may find it taxing to apply their learning in different subjects to a new area and to combine a progression of concepts to form new learning.

The upper primary and secondary school years also combine with physiological changes as the child approaches puberty and moves into adolescence. This stage for many children (and their parent/carers) can be difficult. For the pre-pubertal child with ASD it can be a time of extreme bewilderment and confusion as their bodies will be changing and their hormones will be heralding emotional imbalance. Many children with ASD will appreciate and make use of factual information regarding the onset of puberty and bodily changes; some will benefit from an individually tailored programme for information and training. For those with more severe learning difficulties a concrete, practical and visual strategy will be needed to reinforce the social and moral rules around sexual expression and care of their bodies (e.g. personal hygiene, menstruation). The typical social behaviours of their peers may also need further explanation and exploration, as many people with ASD think literally and will find it hard to extract meaning from such teenage pastimes as flirting with the opposite sex, drawing attention to oneself, deciding what is 'cool' and what is not. It is also a time when peer pressure can be brought to bear immensely on those who do not conform to the 'crowd' and this can lead to ostracism, isolation and vulnerability.

Moving into adulthood

Moving on from the structured environment of school to something unfamiliar which will probably be much less ordered is going to be a source of huge additional anxiety for the person with ASD. Also, the stresses of adolescence are likely to impact more on youngsters with Asperger syndrome, so they can be at an increased risk of other psychological problems (Tantam, 2000). There are narrower choices for youngsters with ASD, and planning needs to begin at an early stage to find out what is available, and whether it is appropriate. The young person may be required to make important but abstract decisions and choices at this stage, when they may still be emotionally quite immature. They may also lack the practical skills to move on to the setting of their choice (for instance, the travel skills to get to work or college, or the independence to go to university) and the teaching of these skills may need to be a priority.

Throughout their life, there will be key transitional stages that will place new social demands on the individual. It is to be expected that such demands will affect the behaviour of the individual at times and they will have different support needs at these points. The majority of individuals with ASD develop some coping strategies as they mature, and so may appear deceptively to be more competent socially than they actually are. With any individual on the spectrum, it should be assumed that they are facing enormous social challenges on a daily basis and that they will need sensitive support to help them manage the pressure and anxiety caused by this.

Key transitions as the young person moves to adulthood

Below is a list of transitions that the young person may encounter as they reach, and progress through adulthood:

- Further or higher education – Colleges and universities are generally much larger and far less structured than the school environment. Students are given the rights and responsibilities of adults, which place increased social pressures on the student with ASD, both to take responsibility for their own studies and to cope with fellow students, who may be less controlled than at school.
- Work placement or employment – Whether this is a sheltered/supported placement or a paid position, the work environment has a specific set of social rules that apply.
- Residential placement – Those individuals with living support needs will often find themselves in a group home or other communal living placement, where they are expected to share space with strangers. Adult care settings are not led by the curriculum and are often less well funded than educational provision. This can mean that there is less scope for individual work and the person will find themselves more often in shared environments.
- Supported living or independent living – Conversely, the more able person may find that they are not entitled to support and are expected to live alone and cope independently. This can lead to an extremely isolated lifestyle, where the onus is on the individual to maintain all social contact. Social exclusion is a significant risk here, which can lead to de-skilling and extreme social anxiety. It is likely that at different points in their life, the individual will move between the common options outlined above, and unfortunately, there may well be times when the individual has no constructive activities available to them, either as a result of exclusion or lack of availability.

In supporting individuals to develop social skills, it is worth considering how this may be experienced by the person concerned. You are attempting to teach the individual an area in which they are naturally weak and are likely to have had bad experiences. You can anticipate therefore that their reactions will include:

- high levels of anxiety and fear
- resistance to trying new things
- strong feelings about activities or areas where they have had bad experiences in the past
- sensitivity to criticism, which may verge on paranoia if they feel someone is reacting badly to them.

These reactions are understandable, and to counter them:

1. Tap into natural strengths and interests so that the activity is enjoyable.
2. Ensure that the activity is meaningful, so that individuals are well motivated.
3. Make outcomes and your own expectations explicit so that the individual understands what is expected.
4. Provide opportunity for practice, so that the skill can be developed.
5. Check and re-check that positive reinforcement is built into the activity and that there are explicit signals and feedback to indicate that the individual is doing well – in the area of social skills, the natural response is often disapproval for an inappropriate behaviour, whereas appropriate behaviours receive no reaction at all. The person does not get the feedback that they have behaved appropriately and so will be less likely to repeat the behaviour.

CASE STUDY

The following case study illustrates how social skills can be effectively and positively taught.

Daniel has ASD and moderate learning disability. He has no speech but understands both speech and sign. He can become highly anxious in public places and in the past this has led to him displaying problem behaviours. Risk assessments at the time dictated that he could not access the community with less than 2:1

staffing, severely restricting his opportunities. The ability to be calm in public has been identified as an essential social skill for Daniel's quality of life.

Following the template above, a teaching opportunity was developed:

1. Daniel's favourite meal is spaghetti bolognaise and he enjoys 1:1 attention, so it was decided he should be supported 1:1 to cook this meal once a week – ENJOYMENT
2. As a natural precursor to the cooking activity, a shopping trip was planned to buy the ingredients. This trip would include Daniel choosing the dessert for that day, which was considered an additional motivation that would give variety each week – MOTIVATION
3. Photographs were used to create a timetable of tasks for the activity – these were put in a small album in chronological order which Daniel was given to carry. Each week the album was used as a prompt for the different stages of the activity, so that there was a clear, regular routine – CLEAR OUTCOME
4. The shopping trip and lunch became a regular weekly activity, initially using the same shops. This meant that Daniel and his supporter met the same assistants each week, who began to speak to Daniel as they became familiar with him. Daniel responded well to this, as it happened gradually and he had time to build his confidence – OPPORTUNITY FOR PRACTICE
5. Support staff were careful to highlight the positives to Daniel, both in terms of planned outcomes, such as Daniel purchasing ingredients from the assistants himself, and incidentals such as the developing familiarity with assistants. Photographs were taken regularly as reinforcers and Daniel was encouraged to create his own wall collage using these – POSITIVE FEEDBACK

Daniel was very proud of this and in fact photography developed naturally as an interest. This itself became a motivator for him to access the community, opening up other, new opportunities for him which staff would never have anticipated.

REFLECTIVE OASIS

Can you identify some of the social coping strategies used by the person you know?

How can you make the social environment less challenging and more rewarding for the person concerned?

Points to remember

- The triad of impairments has an impact throughout life.
- The infant with ASD can appear passive and unengaged.
- School can be a very confusing place for children and young people with ASD.
- Transition from one service to another needs careful planning.
- Teach turn-taking.
- Have clear rules and expectations.
- Provide opportunities for skills to be learnt in different settings.

Overview of current research

This chapter will look at some tried and tested approaches, strategies and interventions that have targeted social behaviours, the development of social skills and social understanding.

Over the last 10–15 years, new strategies and approaches have been developed, predominantly for use at school or at home. Quite often the approach will address one area of the triad of impairments – language and communication, for example, is well served by the Picture Exchange Communication System (Bondy and Frost, 1994). Few approaches seem to target the social differences manifest in ASD. Efforts of parents/carers/practitioners may be on modelling and teaching particular social conventions – hand-shaking, having a ready universal greeting, teaching good manners. However, if the individual with ASD does not understand social situations, or cannot differentiate when to say 'Hello, you look lovely today' (fine for Mum but not for the unknown woman in town) then learnt sayings and rote responses may just highlight individual differences.

Rogers (2000) has called the differences around social interaction as 'perhaps the most defining feature of autism'. The development and improvement of social skills has a correlation with a positive long-term adjustment (Ozonoff and Miller, 1995). Wimpory et al. (2000) highlight the social interaction and communication difficulties of children with ASD who are under 2 years old often have the absence of prerequisites to interaction of pointing, showing, attracting attention. Early difficulties in establishing a means of communication will have an impact upon the development of social behaviours and widen the gap between children with ASD and their peers.

Social stories

Social stories (Gray, 1994, & 2000; **www.thegraycenter.org**) can help the individual with ASD learn how to handle certain situations. The strategy helps to explain the social situation and tries to give both the perspective of other 'players' and their expectations of the individual. The target situation or response is woven into a story with the individual with ASD at the centre and is told either in first or third person. With the individual central in the story, the load on comprehension is lightened because the story is explicit. Gray suggests that certain types of sentences should be used in the story:

- Descriptive: To define what happens – 'where', 'why' and 'what' statements. Occasionally use the word 'sometimes' to give flexibility.
- Directive: To state the desired response in a given situation and phrased in positive terms. Better to use terms like 'will try' rather than 'will do'.
- Perspective: To describe the behaviours, e.g. feelings, reactions, responses of others involved in the situation.

Ideally the story should include between two and five descriptive and perspective statements for every directive statement, so that it does not become a list of dos and don'ts.

Social stories involve interaction with and reinforcement by others. Usage must be consistent, so that if an inappropriate behaviour does occur, the story can be used to cue appropriate behaviour. Involve older individuals and more able children in the writing process. A joint decision can be made to target something that is causing problems and where it is most likely to occur. It may be necessary to involve other people in order to give consistency of usage or approach. Chalk (2003) highlights how social stories have been used well in an adult care setting.

Extra information may be given by illustrating the story with drawings and photographs. The story needs to be used regularly and monitored carefully to gauge whether it has brought about a change in understanding or behaviour.

Example

Shutting the door in the toilet

When I go to the toilet at home I keep the door open

My family knows that it is me

When I go to the toilet in a public place, like McDonald's, I keep the door open

This means that other people can see what I am doing

Other people like to be private when they use the toilet, so they shut the door

They do not want anybody to see what they are doing

Going to the toilet is a private thing to do

I will try to shut the door every time I use the toilet.

Social sentences

Social sentences can be used to help those with ASD to make sense of situations. Short information bites, reminders or prompts are delivered quickly and effectively.

Example

Sometimes people don't answer when you talk to them

Possible reasons:

Maybe they…

did not hear you

weren't paying attention

were busy

Decision/outcome:

I can forget about it, maybe they will answer later.

Social skills groups

Nita Jackson (2002) discusses the valuable social skills group she attended, set up by Essex Social Services with seven young people with Asperger syndrome and four teachers. Nita describes the teachers as friendly and open-minded, who encouraged the group to express themselves. Some social groups, like Nita's, are highly structured and follow a specific issue, e.g. personal space, interrupting, bullying and avoiding danger. Other groups are discussed in Chapter 5. Some schools are now establishing after-school clubs and Saturday clubs for pupils with ASD. When organising leisure activities, a risk assessment may be needed.

CASE STUDY

Social group

A local voluntary sector organisation created opportunities for young adults with Asperger syndrome to develop their social skills. Five individuals had been identified who wanted to improve their skills. The typical profile was of socially interested individuals who became anxious in social situations.

1. Regular social activities were established: group activities with one or two support staff, in natural local settings, such as pubs, restaurants, cinemas, etc.
2. Activities were selected by group members to reflect their own interests.
3. Targets were not set; enjoyment and a relaxed atmosphere were important. Basic ground rules covered behaviour and support for one other; to encourage consideration of the way they inter-acted. As the group became established and members devel-oped confidence, they were encouraged to take responsibility for arranging their activity.
4. As different members preferred different types of activities, and were encouraged to try out new things from time to time, there were opportunities for practice in real situations.
5. Informal feedback was offered during each activity. Group mem-bers were encouraged to support and praise one another. The group was encouraged to reflect on both their individual and shared achievements in occasional meetings. Any incidental outcomes were explicitly stated. For instance, a man with an interest in cinema became confident enough to join a local film group – an outcome of his experiences.

Circle of friends

A circle of friends (CoF) is a social support mechanism that helps the person with ASD to feel less isolated at break times and lunch times, and during group or team work tasks. CoF has the purpose of assisting young people to adapt to settings (Whitaker et al., 1998). A circle usually consists of six to eight volunteers who meet on a regular basis with the 'focus person' and an adult/practitioner. The circle has three main functions:

- offering encouragement and recognising success
- identifying difficulties, setting targets and devising strategies for achieving targets
- helping to put these ideas into practice.

In setting up a CoF in school, it will be necessary to gain support and agreement from the 'focus person' and parents; meet with the whole class to recruit volunteers; gain agreement from the parents of the volunteers; and organise weekly meetings. When an adult is the focus, practitioners need to ensure that their wishes and feelings are respected and that parents/carers are consulted. Permission may not be needed if the focus person agrees and is over the age of majority.

An individual with ASD may choose to make their own CoF with 'like-minded' others. Research by Frederickson, Warren and Turner (2005) found that any changes were in the attitudes of the peers of the target child, rather than any change in the target child's behaviours. While this may make the peers more accepting of the child, the long-term benefits of an attitude change could be negligible. They believe that running concurrent programmes to focus on social behaviours and problem-solving may improve social acceptance and inclusion.

Social Use of Language Programme (SULP)

SULP (Rinaldi, 1993) aims to increase functional language by focusing on pragmatics, which deal with the meaning of words. Learning about pragmatics helps people with ASD to:

- understand the meaning in conversation
- use features of interaction such as facial and non-verbal communication

- develop conversational structures
- examine the wider influence of communication – social situations, backgrounds, attitudes.

The SULP programme makes use of strong visual and graphic stimuli, and deals with age-appropriate issues and everyday situations. It provides opportunities to practise new skills and concepts via motivating activities or tasks. Versions of SULP cover skills for the very young – eye contact, awareness of personal space – through to story packs for teenagers and adults, dealing with examples of appropriate social skills like paying attention to your listener when they are speaking. The programme is often something that speech and language therapists (SALTs) have been trained in.

Behavioural programmes

Work by Davis et al. (1994), Belchic and Harris (1994), Koegel et al. (1992) and LaLonde and Chandler (1995) has used behavioural methods to teach interactional and conversational skills. Davis et al. used a series of rapid requests of child-favoured activities followed by a request to interact. They reported an increase in unprompted initiations and extended interactions which were transferred to other settings.

Belchic and Harris worked with children aged between 4 and 5 and taught them how to initiate and maintain social interaction with their peers, resulting in more time in interactions. Koegel et al. used a reinforcement strategy to encourage interactions but once the reinforcement was removed, the interactions decreased. Many people with ASD do not find social interaction worthwhile for its own value. LaLonde and Chandler used a five-point framework to teach conversational skills with criteria for mastery of each skill area. Increases were in the amount of time spent in interactions and the amount of spoken language for some.

The use of behavioural techniques and their efficacy has been the subject of long and intense debate (see critiques of the Lovaas approach). Their limitations lie in the motivation of the person with ASD in skills that do not come easily. Where extrinsic reinforcement is used (often food), progress can be rapid but maintenance can fail once the reinforcement is removed. Social skills which require discernment and interpretation, and are socially governed often cannot be taught in a universal, rote fashion because every taught response needs a judgement on when and whether to use it.

Using adult-assisted learning

These approaches use significant adults in the lives of people with ASD, such as parents and carers, as opposed to professionals. Work by Dawson and Galpert (1990) trained parents in specific interaction approaches with their young child, and reported an increase in social initiations and tolerance. Krantz and McClannahan (1993) used play scripts to teach play skills and found that as the scripting content diminished, the unscripted initiations increased. Older children had similar results (Stevenson et al., 2000).

Using peer child training

Children with ASD may make and receive fewer social interactions, and make fewer responses in a shorter length of time than their peers, but work by Potter and Whittaker (2001) shows that we often do not pay attention to the times and different ways in which they try to initiate. For example, inappropriate or unwanted behaviours (see Chapter 4) are often a means of communicating something that urgently needs to be brought to our atten tion. CoF (Whitaker et al., 1998) is one way of using peer child training in social interactions, and work by Mundschenk and Sasso (1995) and Lord and Hopkins (1986) used similar peer priming approaches to CoF. One of the advantages of using peers to train the child with ASD is that they are 'on the spot' and have consistent and continuous access to the child. Laushey and Heflin (2000) used a peer buddy system to increase social interactions with young pre-school children.

Strain and Danko (1995) suggest that the gains apparent in using peer child training could be generalised to the home environment, with parents/carers teaching siblings and relations how to interact effectively with the child.

Social play record

The social play record (White, 2006) is a tool that helps practitioners to assess and develop social play. A comprehensive data collection builds up a holistic social picture of the child and their current skills in a variety of contexts. It gives a range of ideas and opportunities by using worked examples of how to understand the individual and take their present skills forward, by assessing the situation, alongside suggested interventions. The use of self-assessment sheets helps the child to have a voice in outlining their own social preferences, instead of a prescriptive, practitioner-led interaction.

Social skills groups for children and adolescents with Asperger syndrome

The book by Kiker Painter (2006) includes practical sessions to enable the young person with Asperger syndrome to work through social skill essentials, such as understanding tone of voice, the range of emotions, phone conversational skills. The aims and rationale for each taught session are given as well as the equipment needed. Notes for the parents as well as the teacher are included, aiming to make generalisation of skills learnt in each session straightforward.

Computer-assisted learning (CAL)

There has been considerable interest in the area of computer programs using emotion recognition or virtual situations. Some have focused on the development of social skills (Silver and Oakes, 2001; Beardon, Parsons and Neale, 2001) and others have looked at developing areas such as problem-solving (Bernard-Opitz, Sriram and Nakhoda-Sapuan, 2001). This work has capitalised on the common aptitude that people with ASD have for information technology. CAL may remove unpredictability and the need for social interpretation with peers. Smith (2003) reports that CAL research has demonstrated skill-gains in:

- reading and communication skills
- vocabulary acquisition
- fundamental learning.

Baron-Cohen (2003) has also produced a computer-based programme to help people with ASD to study emotion and learn how to interpret facial expressions and vocal tone.

There is a number of websites organised by and for people with Asperger syndrome which offer peer support through Internet chat rooms, and the value of peer support can be immense for this potentially isolated group (Sainsbury, 2000).

Video-assisted learning

Most homes and schools now own a video and/or digital camera to capture instant and spontaneous images. Lewis (1999) had a permanently mounted video camera in her classroom to record events during the day. Using video footage, streamed through computer or played back on a recorder, helped one boy with ASD analyse his interactions with others and make a hypothesis on how and why others reacted as they did. Charlop and Milstein (1989) used a recording of simple and appropriate conversational exchanges with three children as a way of teaching models of acceptable interactions. Using footage from TV 'soaps' with individuals with ASD can help to analyse social events and accompanying behaviours, modes of speech, etc. There is some support for use of these techniques as they focus on visual learning, which many with ASD are said to favour (see Plimley and Bowen, 2006a, for further discussion).

Points to remember

- A number of strategies has been developed to help individuals with ASD with social communication and interaction.
- It is useful to consider strategies such as social stories, social sentences, social skills groups, circle of friends and the Social Use of Language Programme.
- Social Play Record is a tool used by practitioners to assess and develop social play.
- Other strategies that help may involve adults, peers, computers or videos.

4

Analysing behaviour

This chapter emphasises the importance of analysing behaviours and finding the meaning behind them. It examines a number of strategies that can be used to pinpoint the triggers for behaviour. 'Challenging behaviour' may occur because an individual with ASD is under extreme stress.

A word about behaviours

For many, the typical picture of a person with ASD will have the accompaniment of behaviours that are often far more extreme and/or inappropriate than is acceptable. Many people associate extreme behaviours with the autistic spectrum, but in fact there are no typically 'autistic' patterns of behaving. Most behavioural outbursts stem from a challenge to the comfort and feeling of security of the individual. They sometimes arise after a supreme effort of control, only to have a 'straw that broke the camel's back'. We have moved away from looking at the behaviours and trying to 'treat' them. Terminology has changed from negative connotations of violence and aggression towards a transactional point of view of behaviours that challenge – they challenge us to do something about them. We no longer seek to control the person by restraint, punishment and/or drug regimes.

Overview and construct of behaviour

'Challenging behaviour' has become part of our everyday speech as a description of aggression, violence and destructive behaviours. The emphasis on ownership has changed, away from behaviours being the responsibility of their 'owner' to the onus on parents/carers and practitioners to take on the challenge. Cumine et al. (1998), Zarkowska and Clements (1998) and Whitaker (2001) put the responsibility on practitioners to analyse the reasons for the behaviour and devise a means of de-escalation. By documenting the series of events and behaviours that has taken place, our focus should be on the function of the behaviour for the person who is being 'challenging'. Often, it is the need to escape a situation causing distress or the sensory overload it represents. Repeated actions are often a way for them to regain control over a situation by producing a predictable set of responses from us.

Lawson (2000) says the following responses are typical reactions to an overload of sensory stimulation:

- pacing up and down
- covering ears with one's hands
- screaming
- excessive spinning or rocking of one's body
- loud verbalisation
- total withdrawal
- aggression
- head banging
- self-injury
- irritation.

(Lawson 2000, pp. 78–79)

'Challenging' responses that might diminish stress include:

- asking the same questions repeatedly
- rocking vigorously
- flapping
- tapping
- absconding or removing oneself from the setting
- jumping up and down.

The term 'challenging' is used because the behaviour is not within our accepted range of responses. Extreme and repetitive challenging behaviours, which the person finds hard to move on from, become 'ritualistic', in our terms. We feel an urgency to control or extinguish these types of behaviour because of their severity and damage to the individual, others or the setting. Where a team is involved, the onus is often on them to 'deal with the behaviour'. Intervention can be ineffective because the behaviour is not responded to in a consistent way. Effective intervention involves working together with the person and important people in their life, to teach socially acceptable alternatives, including articulating the cause of their discomfort.

Finding out the function of the behaviour

Ask yourself the questions 'what function is the behaviour fulfilling for the individual?'; 'does it get the individual removed from an activity they don't want to be in'; 'does it get rid of people they don't like?' Avoid assuming that the behaviour is deliberate and targeted. Extremes of behaviour are almost certainly a means of communicating something for the individual with ASD. We have to pay attention to the message it conveys or the behaviour will not be modulated. Consider the following factors:

- The perceptions of important others – has the behaviour happened over a long time, does it occur with them, what is their response?
- The perception of the individual – are they aware of its impact, do they know how it looks from the outside (video use or digital images)?
- Do they want to find a less stressful response?
- Re-frame the way the behaviour is viewed by us or others. Is it always viewed as naughty or awkward? Use the behaviour as an opportunity to put something right.
- How could it be shaped into something more acceptable and appropriate?
- A positive approach to the person and their behaviour is more humane and likely to achieve a better result.
- Teach an acceptable way of achieving the same outcome result, e.g. a signal that lets us know stress levels and tolerance are OK or near to explosion.

A graphic way of looking for the message in the behaviour is to put a stick figure in the centre of some drawing paper and draw a series of thought bubbles around them.

Bubble 1 – an accurate description of the behaviour

Bubble 2 – three things that the behaviour might be communicating in the individual's own 'voice', using 'I' statements

Bubble 3 – the checks that you might need to make in order to ascertain the frequency of the behaviour, the places where it happens, the people who are present, whether the person is having an off-day or is potentially sick

Bubble 4 – the strategy/ies that can be tried in order to give the person a more acceptable way of communicating the message at the source of the behaviour.

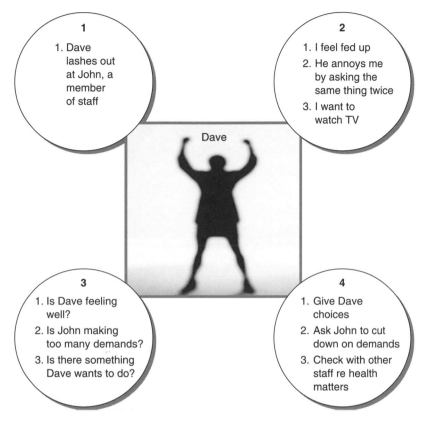

FIGURE 4.1   Analysing Dave's Behaviour

CASE STUDY

Robyn had a very effective way of letting other people know when to back off. She bit them. No matter how quick the staff members and other service users were, Robyn usually managed a strong bite at their forearms. This led to an injured and wary staff team and worried carers of her peers who did not feel that Robyn 'should be accommodated here.' Attempts at trying to extinguish the biting, including time away from the group; removal of watching her favourite video; protective armwear for the staff; a firm 'No' in her face and a period of exclusion had failed to remove this response from her repertoire. A key worker decided that perhaps Robyn would just like more personal space. Often the staff group closed in around her when the behaviour was at its worst, which intensified the damage done. The key worker gave Robyn a symbol to use that everyone could understand. It showed a raised palm of a hand with 'Go away please' written underneath. The staff team and service users were informed that if Robyn showed the card then they were to back off without argument. In under a fortnight, the biting response had diminished in frequency from three or four times per day to once or twice per week because Robyn had found a new means of communicating what she wanted.

By looking at the communicative function of Robyn's behaviour, the key worker was able to replace something that was challenging, damaging and lowering of everyone's morale by an acceptable way of communicating.

REFLECTIVE OASIS

Try looking at a 'target' behaviour for its message, using the graphic method or by analysing its communicative function in another way.

How does framing the situation in the voice of the person 'doing' the behaviour help us to see their perspective?

What other situations may the person with ASD be trying to give you a message about?

Interventions that punish

Behaviorist theory of the 1960s and 1970s advised intervention in the behaviour, and introduction of a consequence that had an aversive effect (shouting, removal, physical punishment). Practitioners working in care and school environments would be expected to find a way of stopping the behaviour. Use of corporal punishment, which had not been made illegal, may have also been a sanction for bad behaviour.

It is a mistake to try to extinguish (remove) behaviours without teaching a more acceptable replacement activity. To punish and/or use aversive practices in response to the behaviour will only teach the person anxiety, fear and/or discomfort. The outcome may be an element of conformity, but the person will not have a 'replacement' that gives the same message. Conformity can become a learned behaviour. The individual with ASD may conform just to avoid further stress.

Using observation and recording for incidents of challenging behaviour

The nature of some behaviours that individuals with ASD manifest may leave us feeling demoralised and de-skilled. This is especially true if the results are injury and harm to those around them. An adult with ASD may engage in behaviours which might have been endearing as a youngster – wanting to sit on an adult's lap, interest in people's clothing or jewellery, conducting an imaginary fight with an imaginary opponent to defuse stress. Transpose those behaviours into adult-hood and a stranger witnessing the behaviour could be very frightened. It is imperative that some behaviours, appropriate in childhood but inappropriate in adulthood, are tackled early with the aim of replacing the behaviour with some-thing that will be more socially acceptable, whatever the age.

Quite often, those who live with and care for the individual with ASD claim to have 'tried everything' in attempting to shape behaviours. Their theory may be that it is 'learned' or 'copycat'. Our constructs and attempts to intervene are influenced by those beliefs. To analyse them, we must deter-mine how, why and when these behaviours occur. Having a structure to recording and observation is needed.

The following systems of record keeping are retrospective, not contemporaneous – they are filled in after the sequence of events has occurred. They should be completed as soon as possible after the incident, to ensure accuracy. A discussion of the advantages of each model appears in Plimley and Bowen (2006b).

ABC records

One of the most familiar retrospective recording systems is the use of 'ABC charts' (Presland, 1989), with the three letters standing for:

A – Antecedents – events leading up to the incident

B – Behaviour – factual record of behaviours observed

C – Consequences – events after the behaviour.

Retrospective recording once the incident has finished helps to identify and analyse behaviours that are both challenging and persistent. Data collected using the ABC method should be done over a short period before a thorough analysis. ABC recording is very useful in helping to pinpoint specific antecedents or consequences, like the removal of the individual from the situation.

STAR

Zarkowska and Clements (1998) focus on the significance of the setting. The STAR approach was first developed for people with severe learning difficulties (including those with ASD) and looks at:

S – Setting – where the challenging behaviour took place, including presence of others and the activity

T – Trigger – the events/sequence of actions that may have set the behaviour off

A – Action – what the person actually does

R – Results – the aftermath of the behaviour and what function of the behaviour is for that person.

The STAR approach aims to gather factual information. It helps us to consider other factors which may be influencing the behaviour of a person with ASD.

8 STEP (Whitaker, 2001)

The eight steps begin with the collective decision of where to start, which is often the hardest thing to do if you are working as part of team. The steps conclude with the decision of how to pre-empt incidents, how to teach new skills and behaviours and how to make the function of the behaviour less of a reward for the individual.

To pre-empt a major escalation, Whitaker (2001) suggests trying:

- removing the identified trigger
- responding to the behaviour as a communication

- distracting
- reminding the person of a reward
- reminding the person of 'rules'
- providing an opportunity to 'chill out'
- restating the request
- making a small change to request/scale it down
- calming things down

If the incident continues to escalate, ensure the personal safety of others, by:

- making the environment safe
- removing others, if needed
- requesting or calling for assistance
- making your response low key (neutral body language, no eye contact)
- using a physical intervention with other trained staff.

The adrenaline produced by the event may take up to two hours to subside. This is why, when things become calmer, they can suddenly flare up again. Give the individual time, without pressure to regain their own control. Once the recovery phase begins, remember to:

- give space
- try to restore normality to the situation
- calmly restate your demands
- talk the situation through, if possible
- seek support from other staff with the individual and also for yourself.

REFLECTIVE OASIS

Using one of the three recommended approaches, collect data over a week on a behaviour that is perceived as challenging.

Use the data to:

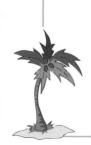

- analyse the function of the behaviour
- discuss with others
- decide how to approach future incidents
- ensure that you have interpreted the function of the behaviour accurately.

Sometimes inappropriate behaviour in a public place can be misinterpreted and lead to prosecution. For example, inappropriate touching or questioning could be misinterpreted as harassment (though not intended). Issues relating to behaviours which may cause offence and lead to involvement with the criminal justice system are explored in depth in Chapter 6.

Finally, strategies that react only to the behaviour (e.g. physical intervention) should be short-term. But remember that 'challenging behaviour' is not simple or speedy to change.

- Look for other reasons for challenging behaviour – is it illness, poor sleeping patterns, diet, lack of communication skills?
- Teach replacement skills alongside ways to identify the build-up of tensions.
- Teach ways in which they can effectively calm themselves – counting to 10 or using de-stressing toys – stress balls, etc.

Above all, treat the behaviour as a form of communication – if the person could successfully articulate what they felt, what would they be saying ?

Points to remember

- Behaviour may be a vehicle for alerting us to the fact the individual with ASD is under extreme pressure. It is important to find the function of the behaviour.
- It is sometimes useful to look at behaviour in a graphic way (Figure 4.1).
- Interventions that punish or try to extinguish behaviour are best avoided.
- ABC, STAR and Whitaker's 8 STEP Plan are useful tools to analyse behaviour.

5

Positive role models

This chapter looks at a wide range of role models that could be used to develop social skills of individuals with ASD.

In an era where the buzz words are 'inclusion' in education and 'social inclusion' in society, and where services strive to offer 'normalised' experiences, we need to look carefully at how these philosophical trends will impact upon people with ASD. It is often assumed that people with ASD will form homogenous communities if they are educated and/or accommodated together. There is no reason to assume that people with ASD will 'fit together' any more readily than anybody else, because each person with ASD, like the general population, is an individual. Grouping people together by dint of a disability is an erroneous assumption which may not benefit either the service users or their carers or staff. Resources can be focused and sourced to suit the group of people with a disability better, but in terms of making a better community, this does not necessarily follow.

Parents and carers often believe that by placing their child within an inclusive school, they will have more positive role models to copy. Although people with ASD are often thought to be poor imitators, in many instances they do copy the behaviour of others. However, the role models that they choose may not be the most positive ones. Good behaviour in schools, although an expectation, does not always have its rewards. Sometimes it can get you noticed by being praised or picked out in front of the whole school, but these are not always the most positive rewards for a person with ASD. Those who misbehave with spectacular results – removal from class, missing a surprise treat or suspension from school – might be the more attractive prospect for imitation from the point of view of a person with ASD.

Sometimes staff and carers have to be more strategic in their placement of role models in order to help the person with ASD both to learn and practise appropriate social skills and to give them socially positive experiences.

Circles of friends (Whitaker et al., 1998)

This strategy (outlined in Chapter 3), is one way of widening the social circle of the individual with ASD. The CoF can help to teach young people age-appropriate skills and behaviours. CoF can broaden the individual's social repertoires and open up an acceptance of new social events, where parents and families have failed.

Buddy system

Emerging work seems to suggest that appointing peer buddies to assist at difficult social times in school (assemblies, playgrounds, lunchtimes) may help to foster inclusion of children with Asperger syndrome (AS), (Mastralengo, 2005; Myles, 2001). This strategy may need the enlisted help of several buddies in order to keep the support going, in a similar way to CoF, as a sole buddy may find it hard to sustain the daily demands of supporting a peer with ASD.

Peer mentoring

Using the skills of the individual with ASD to provide support for others gives recognition to their strengths and can help to work on the reciprocal process of inclusion. It will give the person with ASD a socially valued role within the setting or community. Supporting younger or less able pupils in school and mentoring can be an effective role. Strengths such as maths, reading and IT abilities, as well as leisure skills – chess, video games, special subject collections – may well fulfil this mentoring role (Szatmari, 2004). This can also be continued into adult life where the person with ASD can fulfil a socially valued role in their community, such as computer technician, tax return form assistance, organising bridge games or community historian.

Looking at strategies and mechanisms that can help to support adults with ASD, the Autism Human Rights Charter formulated by Autism Europe (1992) highlights four basic principles:

- rights
- independence
- choice and
- inclusion.

These are also echoed in the White Paper (DoH, 2001) *Valuing People* which aims to improve services for all adults with learning difficulties. The impact of the triad of impairments, especially in the areas of communication and social interaction, may set a boundary on the achievement of these principles. The following strategies have been used effectively with adults with ASD and are only some recommendations of how social supports can be structured.

Circles of support

The principles behind circles of friends also have some resonance in the creation of Circles of Support (CoS) for adults with ASD. CoS can be used to contribute to person-centred planning and open the dialogue between carers, agencies and the individual with ASD (Gold, 1999; Brock 2002; Hatton, 2002). The article by Hatton (2002) highlights an outing that was planned for Tom, a young man in his twenties. The piece takes us through the history of Tom and his relationship with the author, who was a tutor at the local college that Tom attended. His CoS consists of a core group of five people who meet every six to eight weeks. The circle has grown into a supportive network that has helped Tom write important letters to social services, view potential supported accommodation and link up with the Disability Employment Adviser. It has enabled Tom to look at things realistically and to have patience for bigger decisions to be made. The Circles Network (www.circlesnetwork.org.uk) is a national organisation which offers resources, training and information on setting up circles of support and also strategies for introducing person-centred planning, a recommendation of the *Valuing People* (2001) White Paper.

Social groups

A description of a social skills group (Jackson, 2002) appears in Chapter 3. As individuals with ASD mature, they may need other types of social support mechanisms. This is particularly true of the population of people with ASD who are of average or above average intelligence; most typically, if diagnosed, those with Asperger syndrome. Although this group of individuals might be expected to have a wider range of social skills, this may not necessarily be true. Macdonald et al. (1989) have hinted that the higher cognitive ability may give rise to use of different coping and interacting strategies which may serve to disguise true abilities. Barnard et al. (2001) found that many adults with ASD were not achieving the natural attributes that most of us associate with maturity – social circle, gainful occupation, leisure pursuits, community independence, relationships, etc.

For those with good cognitive attributes but few social skills, public perception can often be awry in understanding their needs. Instead of perceiving the person as having a vulnerability because of their lower social skills, sometimes their behaviour and manner can be interpreted as rudeness, arrogance or just being 'very strange'. Often a late diagnosis is given to the more able individual with ASD, by which time they may have built up a reputation within their local community – so understanding and targeted support may continue to elude them.

Some voluntary organisations or health or social service departments have begun to develop social groups for adults with ASD who are capable of living independently or semi-independently within their own community. Such groups arise from the work of Division TEACCH (Mesibov, Shea and Schopler, (2004); **www.teacch.com**) who aim to offer structure and purpose to social meetings in exactly the same way as they recommend for schools and classrooms.

The following case study is a user's account of a social group that has been running successfully for nearly 10 years.

CASE STUDY

What was it like to meet other people with ASD?

I was greatly relieved to find other people like me who had similar difficulties. At my first group meeting we were all given a list of characteristics typical of people with Asperger syndrome and we looked through each point. For instance, not knowing the right thing to say in a social situation – I could always be relied upon to pick the wrong choice of words! The place where we were meeting had their toilets in a different place and I always get lost at times like these – so I went with someone else and we both ended up lost – which was reassuring in a way. After I had been attending the group for a while, I recognized another member in the street. I went up to him and said 'Hi'. He asked me 'How do I know you?' which is something that I have said to strange people over and over again. What a coincidence!

The best thing about meeting with the group is that I socialise, which is something I don't normally do. I don't have to worry about 'doing it wrong', I don't have to cover these things up from other people who do the same. For example, I like twirling and if I felt like doing that at the group, then I could. (With grateful thanks to Pamela Hirsch.)

REFLECTIVE OASIS

How would you go about canvassing interest in setting up such a support mechanism?

What attributes would be needed for people to support adults with ASD in a social setting?

Social valorisation

Ways of giving a social recognition to the person with ASD will help to foster inclusion on a local and community level. The work teams that the TEACCH approach sets up for young people and adults with ASD give those individuals an identity within their own community. Working together with supervisors or job coaches on community tasks, such a litter clearing, gardening, painting and decorating and car cleaning, enables those who cannot work independently to achieve the feeling of a job well done. When the jobs are targeted at helping the community look better or will accomplish tasks that the elderly and infirm cannot do for themselves, social valorisation comes in. This can happen at a much younger age and lower level by giving the child with ASD a responsibility within the classroom, such as pencil sharpening, book tidying, getting out and putting away equipment.

Vocational training

Sometimes the impact of the triad upon an individual's ability to function in social situations can be so marked that vocational training needs to be offered in preference to employment options. In the world of work, attitudes and values have shifted dramatically in the last half-century, and with the decline of many 'traditional' occupations and the competition of cheaper and more reliable manufacturers, many industries have faded from the work landscape. It is no longer a realistic expectation that all people wishing to be employed will be so throughout their lives; nor, once in employment, are there 'jobs for life' any more. In such a climate, some people question whether it is realistic to raise the hopes of individuals with ASD to expect paid employment. Many people with ASD will have skills and expertise in quite defined areas that could be shaped into good vocational skills. The structure of work may also appeal to their need for an organised framework. Howlin and Goode (1998) say that an increasing number of adults can be considered for vocational schemes, as work is still a major way of obtaining status as an adult. It behoves us to think about opportunities for gainful occupation for adults with ASD from school age onwards, rather than to look at barriers.

Finding employment

The world of work can pose a diversity of challenges to the person with ASD. Ranging from needing to learn work-related skills through to interview techniques, the individual may have differing levels of competence and everyone with ASD will have a unique profile.

WORKSTEP

This programme is offered by Jobcentre Plus to people with disabilities that hamper them in finding employment and keeping a job. The programme gives time for job selection and can tap into existing links with local employers or finding sheltered or supported employment. Once a job is secured, support in the workplace can last up to three years.

Work preparation

Again, this is offered by Jobcentre Plus to help people with difficulties to compose appropriate CVs, letters of application and prepare for interview.

Prospects Employment Consultancy

The National Autistic Society is one voluntary organisation that has established its own employment scheme in a small number of areas within

England. The Prospects employment scheme helps and supports adults with ASD to enter full-time employment (Mawhood and Howlin, 1999). It has developed a high level of expertise in working with people with ASD and their employers. They support employers in recruiting and selection processes and they give ASD-awareness training. Originally based in London, they also have offices in Glasgow, Sheffield and Manchester.

ASpire Employment Service

This is offered by autism.west midlands, which serves local authorities in central England. ASpire has a contract for work preparation with Jobcentre Plus. Firstly, each individual with ASD undergoes a comprehensive assessment of needs and then they are invited to attend a selection of taught sessions, aimed at meeting the learning needs highlighted through their assessment. This leads to a Practical Work Skills Programme including a placement in work. Job coaching is offered once the individual has secured a job.

Progress in one area can often lead to positive repercussions in other areas, like self-esteem and greater independence.

Points to remember

- Each person with ASD is unique.
- Individuals with ASD need to have the opportunity to learn and practise appropriate behaviours.
- Strategies that might provide positive role models include approaches such as circles of friends, buddy systems, peer mentoring, circles of support and social groups.
- Preparation, support, advice and vocational training will need to be considered prior to employment.

Criminal justice system and emergency services

This chapter gives an overview of the reasons why individuals with ASD might come into contact with professionals in the criminal justice system (CJS) and the emergency services. It examines their vulnerability to commit crime or be the victim of a crime and gives examples of how some individuals might react in the event of an accident. It offers a range of strategies that might help in these circumstances.

Offending behaviour

Sometimes individuals with ASD might come into contact with the CJS because of the nature of their social difficulties, their trusting and open personality, their particular 'special interests' or their sensitivity to sensory experiences.

Howlin (2006) states that individuals with ASD might be particularly vulnerable to crime for the following reasons:

- A fascination or 'special interest' could be fatal, e.g. fire or poison. Howlin cites the example of a young man who had such an interest in washing machines that he would break into shops and people's houses to examine them.
- A strong dislike such as the sound of a baby crying or a dog barking could lead to an aggressive outburst.

- A lack of knowledge of appropriate and inappropriate touch could lead to accusations of sexual harassment. Individuals may love the feel of a particular texture or material such as velvet and think nothing of stroking the back of the lady in front of them if she happens to be wearing a velvet jacket.
- Unexpected violence and outbursts may be provoked by certain triggers in the environment that are not directly evident.
- A preoccupation with or adoration of an individual could lead to stalking.
- Activities appropriate in childhood can be perceived as inappropriate in adulthood, e.g. picking up or tickling toddlers that belong to complete strangers.

Allen et al. (2006) add to this a vulnerability to get involved in computer crime, property destruction, drug offences and theft.

We asked some teachers of youngsters with ASD what they considered to be some of the major issues. They expressed concerns around the fact that behaviours tolerated in childhood have different connotations in adulthood, e.g. touching, asking inappropriate, highly personal questions, pushing into people and not apologising and temper tantrums or outbursts in public places. One teacher expressed concern over the fact that the youngsters can sometimes be provocative and confrontational. Another mentioned the vulnerability of individuals with ASD to be coerced by neurotypicals into crimes such as petty theft and property destruction.

Davis and Schunick (2002, pp. 45–46) argue that individuals with ASD might come into contact with the police for the following reasons:

- Self-stimulatory and self-injurious behaviour such as hand flapping, pinching self, self-biting, repetitive actions and thrashing.
- Wandering alone, e.g. children dressed inappropriately for the weather wandering alone or darting into traffic. (Here they do point out that some children with ASD are attracted to water and may therefore be especially at risk near pools, ponds and lakes.)
- Peering into windows.
- Turning water faucets on and off.
- Behaviour may mimic drug abuse or mental illness.
- Bizarre or disruptive behaviour such as lining up objects, pica (eating inappropriate objects), toe walking, robotic-like speech.
- Hitting or biting people.

- Involvement in altercations, e.g. they may commit a crime without realising what they have done wrong.
- Suspected child abuse – parents may be restraining the child with what may appear questionable force.

Anti-social behaviour

Sometimes the problems may be exacerbated following a crime because of perceived anti-social behaviour of the individual with ASD. For example, in a situation that involved interaction with a police officer they could:

- behave in an extremely socially inappropriate way
- cause offence without being aware they are doing so
- appear aloof, rude, egocentric or insensitive
- not know how to react to certain unknown situations and other people's feelings
- have difficulty understanding and using non-verbal communication
- not like being touched
- have extreme intolerance to certain sounds and smells or other sensory stimuli
- take things literally
- not be able to understand implied meaning or follow a long set of instructions.

We spoke to a group of youngsters about their experiences with the police. Some of them had found themselves in situations where their social communication had led to misunderstandings. For example, one young man said: 'I have been in trouble and they [the police] thought I was being cheeky but I was just being honest.' When asked by a police officer, 'Do you promise never to do this again?', the young man had answered, 'No I do not know if I will ever do it again.' In his mind, he did not want to make a promise that he truly did not know if he would be able to keep. Another, when asked if he had been involved in a shop lifting incident answered 'Yes'. He had not committed the crime but he had been in the shop at the time when the incident occurred. His interpretation of the word 'involved' was very different from that of the police officer. In short, therefore, individuals with ASD may appear to be behaving in an unco-operative way, when actually they are trying to be as open and honest as they can be.

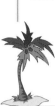

REFLECTIVE OASIS

Think about the children and adults you know who have an ASD. Have any of them ever been in situations where their literal interpretation of language, their 'special interest' or their intolerance levels have led to misunderstandings in a public place?

Strategies that may help

Carrying some form of ID

Some voluntary organisations and family support groups have provided individuals with ASD with an ID card stating potential difficulties.

Feedback on the use of Autism Cymru's Attention card has been very positive:

> *In case I get apprehended wrongly and get stressed.*
> *In case police start asking me questions.*
> *Could use it if you got lost.*
> *I could be in the wrong place at the wrong time and the police might ask questions and get the wrong idea. I would probably react worse than the ones committing the crime. A few years ago I might have hit someone.*
> *If I throw a wobbly in the street, the police would know my problem.*
> *I'd use it in tricky situations or when I am too traumatised to speak.*
> *It will help me stay out of trouble.*
> *Someone with autism or Asperger's could be stuck without this card.*

The scheme has also been welcomed by parents/carers. They feel that the card gives their son or daughter more independence to participate in activities they enjoy, such as travelling by bus, going to football matches or visiting music shops, without their behaviour being misinterpreted.

Sometimes individuals with ASD will take flight when they are feeling under stress – or just because they feel like it. We know of young children who have wandered off in busy streets in big cities, causing their families a great deal of anxiety. One young child even managed to get on a train by himself and was not found until the train reached its final destination. When young children have no language, this creates further problems and often they can be mistaken for having a hearing impairment rather than ASD. The card system may not be entirely appropriate under these circumstances, if the child is unhappy for it to be tagged visibly on to a garment. Wrist bands giving details can be used, but once again only if tolerance levels allow. Davis and Schunick (2002) suggest attaching a silver identity disk to shoe laces where there would be no tactile discomfort and removal would be difficult. They suggest the tag should contain information such as name, address, phone number, behavioural characteristics and contacts.

Social stories (see also Chapter 3)

Social stories (**www.thegraycenter.org**) can be particularly helpful in teaching children how to cope with a range of emergency situations and safety issues such as:

- how and when to use an ID card
- appropriate and inappropriate touching – although such issues would also be an integral part of any sex education programme
- asking appropriate and inappropriate questions
- using a telephone to contact the police and the emergency services
- social etiquette when out shopping or eating
- road safety
- what to do when lost
- using public toilets and changing rooms.

Examining 'special interests'

Many 'special interests' can be quite harmless, e.g. stamp collecting, while others can be potentially hazardous. A youngster with a fascination for fire might be capable of making fire bombs and throwing them out of the window or setting alight a neighbour's property. We recently heard of a young man who had been accused of downloading pornography from the Internet. To him the material was not pornographic or sexual – he just liked to look at pictures of the human body. The 'activity' the bodies were engaged in was completely lost on him. It is important therefore to look at special interests in a wider context. The obvious examples are of course fire, water, poisons and weapons, but other less obvious special interests may also warrant a closer examination, e.g. a strong liking for pulling electronic equipment apart and putting it back together again is fine if the equipment does not belong to someone else!

Looking for triggers

We have mentioned that individuals with ASD might be highly sensitive to certain sensory experiences (see Chapter 1) and this in turn can sometimes lead to aggressive outbursts. If the person you know or work with experiences such difficulties when confronted with particular sounds, sights or smells, try to avoid exposing them to these and teach them strategies that might help them alleviate their stress, e.g. using stress balls, having things to 'twiddle' or fiddle with.

Using the school curriculum

Many issues can be addressed within the curriculum for personal, social and health education (PSHE) and citizenship. Pupils should also be given opportunities to meet a range of professionals from the CJS.

CASE STUDY

A North Wales police officer responsible for working with children and young people attending a residential school for ASD has spent time at the school observing lessons and pupils in order to produce a 12-month curriculum with specific lessons and activities. The programme is delivered as part of the PSHE curriculum and has been differentiated to meet the needs of pupils with ASD and severe learning difficulties. For example, sessions for some youngsters could include familiarisation with a police car and the police uniform.

A visual presentation to older pupils focused on anti-social behaviour. The officer introduced the youngsters to a character called Anti-social Ant and using pictures and photographs showed the damage Ant had caused in the park (drinking alcohol and leaving broken bottles around), on walls (graffiti) and to cars (throwing stones). Ant was also a bully and liked to play loud music. The presentation provoked a great deal of discussion among the group and helped to allay any misunderstandings. The officer then went on to explain about Yellow Cards and Warnings, concepts which can sometimes be difficult to understand. He then discussed Anti-Social Behaviour Orders (ASBOs). The group spent quite some time discussing the implications of the fact that an ASBO could stop them going somewhere, or restrict them from doing something for up to two years.

(With thanks to PC Chris Davies, North Wales Police.)

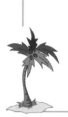

REFLECTIVE OASIS

Do you know a person with ASD who has been in trouble with the police? If so, what were the reasons for this?
Could the situation been avoided?
What strategies have you put in place to ensure that this will not happen again?

Contact with the emergency services

Individuals will also need to be handled very sensitively by professionals within the emergency services. For example, in the event of an accident, their anxiety might be exacerbated by the sudden change in situation, a fear of the unknown, the sounds of sirens, flashing lights and the smell of medication. They can also react very differently to pain and could be in great pain without showing this. In the event of a fire, they retreat if they do not like being touched. Some of the strategies already offered in this chapter will also be useful in helping individuals with ASD to cope with incidents involving fire and ambulance services. Social stories giving an overview of procedures are particularly useful.

A note of caution

Although we have chosen to include a chapter in this book on ASD and the criminal justice system, we would like it to be noted that this does not mean that we are suggesting that individuals with ASD are more likely to be involved in crime than the general population.

Media reports in the UK and abroad can also choose to focus on crime and ASD because it provides a more sensational news item than if the crime had been committed by a 'neurotypical'. It is important that those working and living with individuals with ASD recognise their vulnerability and provide them with the guidance and support they need to avoid contact with the CJS.

Points to remember

- Individuals with ASD can sometimes come into contact with the CJS as both the victims and the perpetrators of crime.
- Strategies such as carrying an ID card and social stories can prevent misunderstandings.

- Individuals should be prepared for any contact they might have with the emergency services.
- Individuals with ASD are no more likely to commit a crime than the general public but they can sometimes be more vulnerable to crime as an offender and as a victim.

7

Moving forward

This chapter gives advice on transition planning from school to further and higher education. It also discusses ways in which individuals with ASD can be prepared for work experience. Person-centred planning is described as a useful tool to prepare for future events.

Transitions

From school phases

A range of resources is available to support transition to new schools (Broderick and Mason-Williams, 2005; Kluth, 2003; Myles, 2001; PAPA, 2003). Positive ideas have been put forward supporting the child with ASD to adapt to a new environment (Plimley and Bowen, 2006a, 2006b). These can be helpful for people with ASD of any age, and include: virtual tours of the new setting on CD-ROM (Cook and Stowe, 2003); a clear visual map of the school, lists of teacher names and room numbers (Myles, 2001); incorporating timetables and room allocations into organisers or Filofaxes for whole-school use; using themes for behaviour expectations (Harpur, Lawlor and Fitzgerald, 2006); having a 'travel card' with lesson reminders and a report by each teacher (Myles, 2001); offering pastoral support that uses letter writing as permanent reminders of issues discussed (Newson, 2000). Jones (2000) suggests the use of a personal passport that records the likes and dislikes, strengths and suggested strategies to help children move around the school environment. This could be adapted for use outside in the community. The Autism Cymru Secondary Forum teachers (2003) offered the following suggestions from their own good practice:

- an A4 topic book with pictures of people and places and vital information on school rules, given a term in advance to a Year 6 pupil
- one afternoon visit per week during summer term
- pupils asked in advance about any worries or concerns
- pupils given a colour-coded plan of school and colour markers placed around school corresponding to different areas for different activities
- using social sentences to state expectations and rules.

These suggestions will transfer to day services, a supported-living environment or other provisions for people with ASD.

From school to further or higher education

Often school will have acted as the central access point for all other support agencies. Once the young person leaves school, there will be no single agency to take on this overarching role. Often the role of co-ordination is down to parents/carers. Co-ordinated multi-agency working is now recognised as best practice. However, the reality for adult services is that systems needed to drive effective collaboration are often not in place. If the young person is of average or above average intelligence, with Asperger syndrome, there is also a persistent lack of clarity about whether they would be the responsibility of learning disability or mental health services. Powell (2002) says that this often results in the individual receiving no service at all. Once a young person reaches adulthood, parents need to be aware that they do not have the same automatic right to information about their son/daughter.

For smooth and successful transition to further or higher education, early planning is absolutely essential. New and unfamiliar decisions will have to be faced by the young person, and they will need the time and space to consider these, and to raise concerns and fears. All parties should be encouraged to consider options holistically. For example, higher education needs to be seen in a bigger picture than an academic option. The demands that will be made on social skills cannot be taken lightly. Most options will need the young person to learn new skills. If these can be identified in advance, and training begun, then the individual will be more successful. To make an informed choice, visiting possible placements and having practical and concrete experience of options is necessary. In considering what subject to study, the individual may choose their strongest school subject. However, they will have to show real aptitude to help them through a graduate programme. Further and higher education offer a huge choice of subjects and this will pose a challenge to any 17-year old. Young adults with ASD will have the combination of fewer social links, be more emotionally immature and less experienced in 'knowing the ropes' to help them decide.

Whether the young person is aiming for a local college or university placement, the difference between that and secondary education will be great. Demands will be made on the young person to multi-task and act on their own initiative (Jamieson and Jamieson, 2004). If the young person begins to struggle early in their studies, they may be overlooked. It is essential to contact student support services early to ensure that potential difficulties are anticipated and planned for. Ideally the referring school can take an active role, as they understand the student's learning needs. Colleges are keen to link with schools to offer taster sessions, and can undertake transitional work.

Arranging work experience in secondary school

A group of secondary teachers who attend Autism Cymru's school forum (2003) were asked what are the key elements in helping youngsters prepare for employment. They suggested the following:

- Good preparation cannot be substituted.
- Prepare pupils in advance – what sort of job they might be interested in?
- Research jobs on the Internet – what is needed to carry out certain jobs (interests, aptitudes, qualifications)? a – allow them to make judgements on suitability.
- Look how best to prepare on both sides – always be honest with the employer; offer awareness training for employees.
- Use visual schedules.
- Teach interview skills, the language of work and the social rules of the workplace.
- Consider and plan for what will happen at break and lunch times.
- Identify a work colleague who could act as a mentor.
- Are there issues around medication?

These points could be a useful checklist prior to a work experience placement.

Planning the programme

Lee (2003) says that transition from school to work can be particularly challenging for individuals with ASD because of their poor communication skills and social behaviours. Stress levels can be heightened and this might result in an individual with ASD becoming withdrawn. Work colleagues might construe this behaviour as aloofness or rudeness and they might choose to ignore the individual.

The transition from education to employment should be gradual and planned over a long period. This includes the young person with ASD having work experience prior to leaving school. Staff at school should liaise with the careers or Connexions service as soon as possible. The young person with ASD, their family and prospective employers must be involved in the process. Employers may welcome the opportunity to have awareness-raising in ASD. The school could play a part in making a short video, emphasising the positive attributes that an individual with ASD can bring to the workplace, but alerting them to potentially stressful experiences in the workplace.

Young people with ASD might find it difficult to cope alone in the workplace and they may need prompting for social cues. It would be advisable for them to have a work-based mentor with a knowledge and understanding of ASD. The mentor could assist the young person with ASD with their timetable and how to prioritise the day. Visual planning would be very useful. Techniques for dealing with stressful situations, such as the card system – yellow card a warning, and a red card for indicating that a limit has been reached. Facilities to enable calming down need to be researched in the workplace. Lunch times and break times in the workplace need to be considered carefully.

Social skills training for the workplace is vital if the placement is going to be a success. Segar (1997) produced a very useful social guide for people with ASD. He says:

> All the same rules apply in the workplace as they do anywhere else but the one difference is that there is something at stake – your job. This means it is extra important to keep a clean slate or you might be the target of scapegoating which is a very nasty threat to your job … if in doubt, keep quiet. This is often seen as a good quality in the office (p. 23).

His advice to those having an interview is: 'You are expected to sit still with your arms by your side'; and 'You are expected to speak clearly and professionally' (p. 23).

Segar suggests that realistic and suitable jobs for people with ASD might be graphic designer, computer programmer, computer technician, research scientist, medical research scientist and architect. He says that people with ASD should avoid jobs that are highly stressful and that involve lots of 'people' skills – for example, salesperson. manager, solicitor, police officer, medical profession or teaching.

Young people at school could collate a portfolio of evidence of positive attributes. This could be used when they have to attend an interview so its contents really emphasise the positives, as the young person with ASD may experience difficulties in communicating openly and directly with an interviewer.

Lee (2003) describes work placement practices in a special school that follows a 'work-related' curriculum. One day per week is spent in the local community, e.g. shops, playgroups, hotels or homes for the elderly. For pupils with greater difficulties, 'in-house' placements are arranged – helping with administrative duties, working with younger pupils, etc. Hesmondhalgh and Breakey (2001) outline a programme for students at a resource base in a secondary school, following a programme of gradual induction into the work experience placement. Students followed the same task for a period of time to help them get accustomed to the changes in circumstances. Tasks were modelled for students and visual prompts such as photographs and picture strips were provided.

A secondary school in mid-Wales with a resource base for youngsters with ASD developed a course known as Future Studies (Jerling, in Plimley and Bowen, 2006a). This aims to show pupils with ASD that everything has a purpose – school, rules, parents, jobs, friends and life. The programme is learner-centred and encourages individuals to examine their own personal strengths and areas for development, what they perceive as opportunities and threats, their short- and long-term plans and career opportunities and options. As part of the programme, pupils are given detailed instruction on job applications, CVs, interviews, college courses, workplace routines and the role of the careers department, teachers and employers. Pupils are prepared for their work experience in a number of ways such as role-play, preliminary visits to the proposed work placement and diary-keeping.

CASE STUDY

SNAP, Cymru's parent partnership service, offers a School Link Volunteer Scheme. School Link volunteers take general enquiries, disseminate general information, support the work of the SENCo, organise parent information sessions, encourage parent-to-parent contact, signpost support to other agencies and involve the wider community in the life of the school.

REFLECTIVE OASIS

Research the opportunities that are available in your area. Is there a School Link volunteer service?

What services do they offer?

If not, how might one be set up?

Person-centred planning

Person-centred planning has required a fundamental shift in the traditional view of care provision, with some practical consequences. The Department of Health's document *Valuing People* (DoH, 2001), which arose from a Social Services Inspectorate Report (1998), says that:

> People with learning disabilities have little control over their lives, few receive direct payments, advocacy services are underdeveloped and people with learning disabilities are often not central to the planning process.
> (DoH, 2001, p. 4)

The guidance given in *Valuing People* on person-centred planning (PCP) stresses the importance of being engaged in 'continual listening and learning' and looking at what is important to the person now and their aspirations for the future. Sanderson et al. (2002) believes that there are five key components crucial to the PCP process:

1. The person is at the centre of the plan.
2. Family members and friends are key partners in planning.

3. The plan shows what is important to the key person (now or for the future). It shows their strengths and what support they need.
4. The plan helps the person to be a part of their community and helps the community to welcome them. It is not just about services. It shows what is possible, not just what is on offer.
5. Things do not just stop when the first plan is written. Everyone involved keeps on listening, learning and making things happen. Putting the plan into action helps the person to achieve what they want out of life (Sanderson et al., 2002, p. 14).

The PCP is a framework that focuses on the person as a whole, not just their behavioural or social needs. It is designed to take the person from where they currently are, to a future that contains their wishes and aspirations, within reason. The contribution of the individual is vital to this process, as are the time and opportunity to enable them to articulate their wishes.

Key areas to be covered, suggested by *Valuing People* (DoH, 2001), are:

- advocacy
- direct payment for care needs
- support for families caring for those with a disability
- improving the experience of transition to adulthood/adult services
- accessing community facilities and services
- increasing opportunities for employment and supported employment
- increasing housing options
- improving access to health services.

The process can take a variety of formats. There are some prescribed formats that follow the five key components outlined by Webb et al. (2002). These are:

- PATH (Planning Alternative Tomorrows with Help) – **www.inclusive-solutions.com/pcplanning.asp**
- Personal Futures Planning – **www.circlesnetwork.org**
- Essential Lifestyles Planning – **www.ELP.net**
- MAPS – Making Action Plans – **www.inclusive solutions.com/pcplanning.asp**

A person-centred plan for Marco, aged 31

Areas considered

- Home
- Work/occupation
- Support
- Leisure interests
- Opportunity for lifelong learning (college)

Home

Marco would like to live in semi-supported housing close to his local town so that he can engage in his special interest of visiting the local art gallery and noting down details of his favourite paintings.

Work/occupation

Marco has a preoccupation with making handwritten lists. In his younger years this has led to cataloguing all of his toys, a database of Wimbledon tennis final scores, listing all of the garden tools in the shed, and the types of T-shirts he has worn over the years.

In more recent times he has developed an interest in Pre-Raphaelite paintings, of which there are many in his local art gallery. He knows about the dates of birth and death of key painters of this period, sites and compositions of many famous paintings and he has catalogued details of the local collection. Marco would like to work in a job where cataloguing and listing are key skills, such as a filing clerk or IT data entry, or work in an art gallery. His local ASD support group has a scheme for job coaching in potential work placements.

Support

Marco comes from a close family and he is the oldest. His parents belong to the local ASD support group. He has two close friends who are very supportive – Megan and Jamie. There is a local advocacy group but Marco or his family have not yet visited them.

Leisure interests

Marco likes walking and rambling. He is surrounded by countryside that takes 10 minutes to reach by bus. He enjoys watching videos and DVDs of Mr Bean.

Opportunity for lifelong learning

Marco went to a painting evening class several years ago, but left after a short while because he did not like the media the teacher wanted him to use. He does have several GCSEs.

Following several meetings and plenty of discussion, with Marco writing down his preferences, a six-month plan of action was agreed (see Table 1).

Table 1   A person-centred plan for Marco, aged 31

ACTIVITY	HOW	WHO
Investigate courses	Get prospectus	Marco
	Talk through courses	Marco with parents
	Arrange visit to providers	Marco
Explore housing options	Contact ASD support group	Marco
	Contact local housing association	Marco and Megan
	Make visits	Marco and Megan
Regular exercise programme	Look at local rambling groups	Marco
	Find companion for daily walk	Marco and Jamie and Fez (Jamie's dog)
	Make approach to rambling club for current programme	Marco and Jamie
	Look at local leisure centre classes	Marco and siblings
Increase art knowledge	Make appointment to meet curator of gallery	Marco
	Do website search	Marco
	Download details of Pre-Raphaelites	Marco
Increase social opportunities	Research local events at library and in local newspapers	Marco, Megan and Jamie

---

REFLECTIVE OASIS

What might a PCP look like for you?

Person-centred planning is being used by service providers for people with ASD. There are some additional things that need to be borne in mind when working with people with ASD:

- Use significant people in their lives, and people that they trust to help with the process.
- Consider how to elicit their views (particularly if they do not have functional communication).
- Consider how, where and when to hold the formal meeting – be flexible.
- Make the format fit their needs – check that the process represents their wishes.
- Make the targets realisable; begin with what they can do and build on that.

Sanderson (2001) sounds a note of warning about the process for all with a learning disability:

> Our approach has to be one of continually asking what it would take to involve people in every aspect of their life, and not just planning. Without this perspective, an investment in finding ways to involve people in a meeting where a plan itself is filed and redundant until the same time next year is futile. This will just add to our list of service abuses of people...

www.valuingpeople.gov.uk/documents/PCPmy-meet.pdf

Points to remember

- Transition across life phases should be considered well in advance.
- Individuals with ASD and their families should be actively involved in the planning.

- Planning for transition from school to FE and HE is crucial and should involve a range of personnel from all sectors.
- Advanced planning and preparation for a work experience placement is essential.
- Person-centred planning is a useful way of considering future needs.

8

Realistic expectations

This chapter stresses the importance of tackling issues and teaching new skills from the perspective of the person with ASD. It considers ways in which we can reduce stress levels by not placing unnecessary demands on individuals and discusses a range of factors for consideration in any teaching and learning programme.

The idea of Cumine et al. (1998) of using an 'Asperger lens' in which to view times of crisis and misunderstanding has proved to be a simple but effective way of helping others to see how different the world is for many people with ASD. The contributions of first-person authors such as Lawson (2000), Grandin and Scariano (1986), Williams (1992), Jackson L. (2002); and Jackson, N. (2002) have enabled us neurotypicals (NTs) to use our empathy to consider how things might be different if the impact of the triad of impairments governed our lives. Tasks that seem straightforward to NTs, like coping with a cancelled appointment or deciding on the order of odd jobs that need to be done around the house, can prove insurmountable if you cannot deal with sudden changes or if you are not able to prioritise. Once we apply an 'ASD lens' to situations that become stressful, we can put ourselves in the shoes of the person with ASD, and support the learning of strategies and simple aids that can help to keep stress on an even level.

If we are trying to support the individual with ASD to achieve their potential at independence, then we need to decide on how to offer that support in the most proactive way. This will mean an assessment of what skill/knowledge-acquisition should be a priority and what features will always be a part of their personality.

This assessment needs to take place in all aspects of our work or lives with the person with ASD. We need to constantly ask the question of ourselves: 'Is this worth making a fuss about?' For example, a child insists on having his ruler, pen and pencil case in exactly the same place on his desk every day, he wraps three fingers around his pen to use it dextrously. The teacher or support worker has two choices:

- Do I intervene and tell him to put his pencil case away because we are doing pasting? Shall I insist on the correct pencil grip?
- This equipment symbolises a structure to him, so it can be left there. He can write and draw accurately and independently, so what will the correct pencil grip achieve that is better than it already is?

These are the types of decisions that we will need to make again and again to weigh up the value of attempting to change established skills and routines, if they are working adequately for the person with ASD. It extends to overreaction and behaviour responses that are inappropriate and unwanted. Sometimes the smaller steps towards achieving their own locus of control can help to avert the bigger blow-ups and traumas. By helping the person to name, recognise and notice their own levels of stress, the dependence on others to intervene can diminish. If you have an unobtrusive, socially acceptable tactic to take the stress out of situations – like going outside for a walk, having a stress-relief toy in your pocket or turning on your mp3 player – then you are responsible for its deployment in times of stress and you do not need others to help you to calm down.

This book and the others in this ASD Toolkit series are aimed at practitioners, parents and individuals with ASD to help increase understanding and identify suitable starting strategies. While identifying many of the differences inherent in ASD, we need to have a 'can do' mentality to find ways through some of the barriers. Historically, those working with people with disability have focused too hard on what cannot be done, without looking at what can be achieved. Legislation and current values are helping to overturn the disabling part of disability and to articulate aspirations, expectations and, above all, ways around the challenges that a disabling condition can present.

We need to take this 'can do' philosophy with us wherever care, education and consideration of those with ASD is offered. Having a realistic approach to what is on offer and can be achieved cannot exist in a vacuum.

For parents and families to have this philosophy but meet with a brick wall of educators who do not share it; for schools and colleges to have this philosophy but to meet resistance when looking for vocational or employment opportunities; for employers to believe in 'can do' only to come up against a 'won't do' care agency, will detract from the achievement and potential realisation of the individual. Fortunately, legislation of recent years, as we have seen, is helping to overturn such defeatist attitudes.

A series of case studies may help to illustrate ways in which potential barriers are being deconstructed to facilitate lifelong learning and independent living ideals.

CASE STUDY

Community Case Study

Jasmine is 20 years old and was diagnosed with autism and learning difficulties at the age of 3, at which time she had developed no speech. As she matured, she developed articulate speech and became fully literate and numerate, and her profile of abilities indicates that she has no learning disability. Although socially interested in others, she is shy and introverted. She lives at home with her mother, on whom she is entirely dependent. She currently has no regular activities outside of those she does with her mother. She has in the past taken college courses designed for students with special needs, but has not been deemed ready to progress from these to either mainstream courses or work placements, so at the moment she seems to have run out of options. During assessment it has been agreed that, for Jasmine to have a wider range of options available to her, the priority at this time is for her to acquire some independence from her mother.

Aim: for Jasmine to learn to travel independently to town by bus.

Enjoyment
Jasmine is interested in fashion and shopping and enjoys eating out. By having a weekly excursion to town, she will have the opportunity to do some regular shopping at stores of her choosing, plus lunch out, so the activity is based on her favourite pastimes.

Motivation
This activity will offer Jasmine some time to indulge her own interests without her mother, and help her develop some of the skills she needs to progress. A college in the town offers courses in fashion and textiles, which Jasmine would love to be able to do. If she is able to develop the skills and confidence to attend the college, her academic abilities would be sufficient for her to get a place on the course.

Explicit outcomes and expectations
The intended outcomes as above were agreed jointly with Jasmine and her mother. Together with their supporter they produced a staged learning plan. Anxieties were running high for both Jasmine and her mother, so it was important that both felt in control of the process. The process was agreed as followed:

Stage 1: Jasmine to travel by bus to and from town, accompanied by her supporter. During this stage, Jasmine would be prompted to stop the correct bus (and stand away from the queue, as appropriate for other buses), buy the tickets and generally take the lead.
Stage 2: Jasmine would undertake the journey shadowed discreetly by her supporter, who would only intervene in an emergency.
Stage 3: Jasmine would undertake the journey independently and be met at the bus stop in town.

Key information (bus numbers, bus stop information, emergency phone numbers) was printed on a laminated credit-card-sized card which could be used with discretion.

Opportunity for practice
Trips were arranged weekly and, since Jasmine's mother was fully involved in the task, she felt confident enough to follow the same format when travelling with Jasmine, so that other opportunities for practice were available.

Positive reinforcement
Regular meetings took place with Jasmine, her mother and the supporter. At this time, each shared their view of how things were progressing, and minor changes were made to the plan where needed. Incidentals were also highlighted: for instance, all agreed that the

increased opportunities to spend time in town have resulted in Jasmine becoming more confident and independent generally. Knowing she would have these opportunities to shop, Jasmine had started to plan particular purchases and save for them. Through regular practice, she had become comfortable at dealing with shop assistants herself, and this meant she was much less anxious around strangers.

The whole process took between six and nine months, with the transition from stage 2 to stage 3 being the most challenging for all concerned. The aims would possibly have been achieved sooner if building work in town had not caused the relevant bus stops to be temporarily moved. Although this caused a regression at the time, it did enable Jasmine to develop other valuable skills in fact-finding and flexibility.

CASE STUDY

Home Case Study

François, aged 4, likes things just so. Any disruption of his familiar environment causes major upset and distress that will continue until his order is restored. His family 'walk on eggshells' around him, unwilling to pose any challenges to his comfort and security. One of François' 'things' is to have the home computer on and accessible at all times. This includes night time when he has been known to get up at 3 am and go and use it. His siblings, who use the computer for school work, often find that their files have been deleted or contaminated by their brother's activities and he is not at all popular! His parents seek advice from their local nursery, who suggest a 'computer on' and a 'computer off' symbol system, which is visually clear and obvious to François. Parents put the symbol and say what it means on the monitor screen. For computer-off times, the whole equipment is disabled via password entry, so that François cannot access it. A diversionary activity is offered to him instead. François was easily diverted during the day by other distractions, but it took longer for him to adjust to night-time controls. The access symbols have also been used for other obsessional activities.

CASE STUDY

School Case Study

Pia did not like anyone at secondary school sharing a desk with her. She made her objections loud and clear enough to disrupt the whole class. However, there were times when she needed to engage in pair and group work to make the best use of her Year 9 studies. Her part-time support worker was able to show Pia on a visual, written timetable when such expectations were going to arise. Pia had a circle of friends group to support her in the school and so she was not short of peers who would voluntarily offer to work with her. Through her circle she had developed a liking for a particular boy in her form and wherever possible she chose to work with him. For group sessions he was able to be an intermediary and suggest to Pia who else they could work with.

CASE STUDY

Adult Case Study

Bill enjoyed his own space. He lived in supported housing, sharing a large house with three other people. He was able to arrange his bedroom to his own taste within the scheme, but he also had strict preferences when it came to communal spaces, including the kitchen. His house sharers, also on the spectrum, would become upset if Bill chose to rearrange kitchen implements or change the contents of each cupboard. This had the effect of de-skilling them as they became disorientated by not being able to find the right things in the same place. Feelings became distraught and hostile towards Bill and there was talk of him having to leave and live by himself. Support staff were able to talk to Bill and give him a simulation of how it feels to have everything moved to new places. With Bill's co-operation, they were able to label cupboard contents with written and graphical symbols so that the storage areas in the kitchen had a function. Bill helped to laminate labels and fix them onto cupboards and had the weekly job of checking through an inventory of items to ensure that everything was in its place.

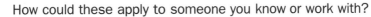

REFLECTIVE OASIS

Think about the issues of independence and realistic expectations raised in these case studies.

How could these apply to someone you know or work with?

Think of proactive ways to increase their levels of independence while paying due attention to the nature of their differences.

Points to remember

- Always try to examine issues from the perspective of the person with ASD (use the 'ASD lens').
- Sometimes insisting on certain approaches to a task can cause unnecessary stress for the teacher and the learner.
- Consider factors such as enjoyment, motivation, explicit outcomes and expectations when teaching new skills.
- Provide opportunities to practise skills.

How to help

This chapter provides the reader with useful strategies that can be used to help individuals with ASD with social communication and social interaction. It draws on ideas and recommendations in previous chapters.

Individuals with ASD, like everyone else, have their own unique personalities. Each will be affected by the triad of impairment in a different way. When using any strategy, this individualism must be borne in mind.

The diagnosis of ASD is a medical one and rests on the presence of the triad of impairments by the age of 3. ASD is a transactional disorder; it is our (NT) interpretation and response that can create the difficulties. People with ASD have contributed greatly to our knowledge and understanding. The opportunity exists for us all to access their work and thoughts (Lawson, 2000; Williams, 1992; Grandin and Scariano, 1986; Jackson, L., 2002; Jackson, N., 2002).

ASD persists through life and although there is no known cure, there are plenty of ways to help alleviate its impact.

- Parent/carers will need to work upon an interaction from their child and build in a functional form of communication.
- Behaviours that challenge will need a systematised approach – to collect data; analyse function and teach replacement responses.
- Always ask whether this behaviour/response will be appropriate for an adult. Teach skills that are appropriate, whatever the age.

- Social stories (Gray, 1994, 2000) help those with ASD to learn how to deal with a range of potentially difficult social situations and acquire some basic social skills.
- Social sentences are a useful tool in helping individuals make sense of a situation or to give them the logical reasons why a situation might occur or a rule might exist.
- The TEACCH approach can be used in a variety of contexts, especially for teaching independence skills. Many individuals with ASD respond to a visual and structured approach to learning.
- People with ASD find many aspects of conversation difficult – they may not be aware when it is their turn to speak or how close they should stand to a person when listening. It is important therefore to develop a teaching programme based on conversational skills.
- Many people with ASD do not find social interaction worthwhile for its own value. The Social Use of Language Programme (SULP) increases functional language by focusing on pragmatics. It makes use of strong visual and graphic stimuli and can help individuals with ASD understand conversation.
- Good role models are important to us all throughout life. For individuals with ASD it may be necessary to have a more strategic approach to the introduction of role models. Individuals with ASD might be assigned to work and play alongside a designated 'neurotypical', e.g. circle of friends, buddy system, peer mentoring.

Often, individuals with ASD are keen to meet up with others who have an ASD. Many such groups have been established by individuals themselves and some of these groups have their own websites and chatrooms, e.g. **www.udel.edu/bkirby/asperger/messageboards.html** or **www.kandi.org/ aspergers/Message_Boards_and_Chat_Rooms/index2.html**. Other groups have been set up by parents, professionals or the voluntary sector.

Such groups can be of immense value to individuals with ASD who might otherwise feel lonely and isolated, particularly in adulthood. They can also be useful forums to teach individuals with ASD appropriate social skills and build their confidence.

Parents have an important role to play in developing social skills and play in younger children. Schemes have been set up to help and advise parents on how they can teach their children new skills especially during the early years. PAPA (2005) runs the Connecting with Autism Project whereby a family is assigned an identified practitioner who introduces them to the

Rainbow Resource Kit. The Kit comprises information booklets, resources, video and a DIY structured activity kit, all of which can be used to make learning with their child fun.

Professionals can use the Social Play Record (White, 2006) to assess and develop play in children with ASD. The strategy emphasises the importance of taking the lead from the child as an active participant.

Computer programs can be useful in teaching individuals with ASD a variety of social skills. Sometimes individuals find computer-assisted learning (CAL) less intrusive. CAL programs examining emotional understanding, e.g. how to interpret facial expression, can be very effective.

Digital and video cameras are invaluable in teaching a variety of skills. They can show individuals how they have reacted in certain situations and be used to provoke discussion. Digital camera images can personalise social stories and bring meaning to a situation. CCTV footage can also be used to discuss what is and what is not acceptable behaviour in a particular environment.

It may not be possible for some individuals with ASD to go directly into employment without help, advice and relevant vocational training. Special interests, skills and expertise can often be shaped into good vocational skills. A number of schemes does exist in an attempt to help in this process, e.g. WORKSTEP, Prospects Employment Consultancy, ASpire Employment Service. Individuals with ASD should be encouraged to be realistic about the type of employment that might suit them. They should keep a portfolio of their positive attributes, which can help at interview.

Individuals with ASD may come into contact with the criminal justice system because of the very nature of their social difficulties. Sometimes they may get into trouble as a result of a misunderstanding, or they may become the victim of a crime because of their trusting and honest nature.

It is also important to recognise that certain behaviours tolerated in childhood may not be so acceptable in adulthood. Forward planning and insight into potential difficulties are essential.

In school, advantage should be taken of the PSHE curriculum to address issues around anti-social behaviour that could cause offence and lead to prosecution. Carers and practitioners should also look for potential triggers that might provoke disruptive outbursts in a public place.

Carrying some form of identification explaining difficulties in social communication and interaction can also be helpful.

Individuals with ASD often have a special interest that continues throughout life. Sometimes special interests can be a useful vehicle for teaching new skills and to encourage social activity, e.g. a chess club or computer club.

They can often be used as a reward and motivation for the acquisition of new skills and can lead to employment.

Unfortunately, some special interests may need closer monitoring as they may lead to difficulties, e.g. fascination with fire, water, weapons, the human body.

Any change – even the slightest – will need to involve an advance warning. Successful transition planning should be prepared well in advance of any move. It must involve a range of professionals, family and most of all, the individual with ASD.

Person-centred planning is an approach that focuses on the future needs of the individual with ASD. It focuses on the person as a whole and not just their behavioural or social needs.

Every opportunity should be given to reduce the stress levels of individuals with ASD. The sensory environment can contribute to stress – new situations, routines, settings, meeting new people or the unnecessary social demands of others. Those living and working with ASD must be highly sensitive to such situations, avoid conflict and create a calming influence wherever possible. It may mean setting somewhere aside as 'a safe haven' for retreat when circumstances become intolerable. Where possible, teach ways in which you might be alerted to stress, e.g. traffic light system, stress alert cards, or provide objects that reduce stress.

It is important to work with individuals to ascertain areas of extreme difficulty and to try to see things from their perspective in finding a solution. Sometimes this might mean a flexible approach to a social situation or a skill acquisition that may not always meet with our own conventions or way of thinking.

Do not try to stop harmless ritualistic behaviour such as rocking or flapping. It may be the only way the individual with ASD has of calming down. Provide an appropriate time and place for this behaviour to take place.

Leisure time is important to everyone. It provides us with the opportunity to relax. Individuals with ASD might need help, advice and support in the pursuit of leisure activities. In some situations, forward planning and the raising of awareness may be necessary, especially if the leisure activity needs to take place in a public centre or club, e.g. swimming, ice dance, judo.

Housing options and the opportunities for lifelong learning will need to be considered in later life. Find out what local agencies and organisations are available to assist.

Any teaching programme must be meaningful for the person with ASD. It must have a reward that is tangible to them, otherwise it will cease to be motivating. Skills are not easily transferred – opportunities will need to be provided for the skill to be practised in a range of situations. Teaching programmes should be designed to facilitate independence.

REFLECTIVE OASIS

Use the pointers above to create an evaluation tool for a person you know with ASD.

What strategies are currently in operation? How effective are they?

Are there any strategies that you have not yet considered?

Is there something that you may need to consider as the person matures?

List your short-, medium- and long-term priorities.

Point to remember

- Although each individual with ASD is unique, most will need some help and support in trying to understand and live happily in a world that can often be most confusing to them.

References

Allen, D., Evans, C., Hider, A. and Peckett, H. (2006) '*Asperger Syndrome and Offending Behaviour*', paper presented by Professor David Allen at Autism Cymru's 2nd International Conference on Autism, Cardiff, 8–10 May. **www.awares.org**

American Psychiatric Association (1994) *Diagnostic and Statistical Manual of Mental Health* (4th edition) *(DSM IV)*. Washington DC: American Psychiatric Association

Asperger, H. (1944) translated by Frith,U. (ed.) (1991) *Asperger and his Syndrome. Autism and Asperger Syndrome*. Cambridge: Cambridge University Press

Autism Cymru Secondary School Forum (2003–6) accessed via **www.awares/.org/edunet www.autismeurope.org/portal/Default.aspx?tabid=30**

Barnard, J., Harvey, V., Prior, A. and Potter, D. (2001) *Ignored or Ineligible? The Reality for Adults with Autistic Spectrum Disorders*. London: National Autistic Society

Baron-Cohen, S. (2003) *Mind Reading: The Interactive Guide to Emotion* (DVD-ROM). London: Jessica Kingsley

Beardon, L., Parsons, S. and Neale, H. (2001) An interdisciplinary approach to investigating the use of virtual reality environments for people with Asperger syndrome. *Educational Psychology, 18(2), 53–62*

Belchic, J.R. and Harris, S.L. (1994) The use of multiple peer exemplars to enhance the generalization of play skills to the siblings of children with autism. *Child and Family Behavior Therapy, 16, 1–25*

Bernard-Opitz, V., Sriram, N. and Nakhoda-Sapuan, S. (2001) Enhancing social problem solving in children with autism and normal children through computer-assisted learning. *Journal of Autism and Developmental Disorders, 31(4), 377–384*

Bondy, A. and Frost, l. (1994) *The Picture Exchange Communication System*. New Jersey: Pyramid Educational Consultants

Brock, S.E. (2002) Group Crisis intervention, in Brock, S.E., Lazarus, P.J. and Jimerson, S.R. (eds) *Best Practices in School Crisis Prevention and Intervention*. Bethesda: National Association of School Psychologists.

Broderick, K. and Mason-Williams, T. (eds) (2005) *Transition Toolkit*. Kidderminster: British Institute of Learning Disabilities

Chalk, M. (2003) Social stories for adults with autism and learning difficulties. *Good Autism Practice Journal, 4(2), 3–11*

Charlop, M.H. and Milstein, J.P. (1989) Teaching autistic children conversational speech using video modelling. *Journal of Applied Behavioral Analysis, 22, 275–285*

Circles Network – **www.circlesnetwork.org.uk**

Cook, L.L. and Stowe, S. (2003) Talk given on Nottinghamshire Inclusion Support Service at Distance education (ASDs) weekend. School of Education, University of Birmingham

Cumine, V., Leach, J. and Stevenson, G. (1998) *Asperger Syndrome. A Practical Guide for Teachers.* London: David Fulton

Davis, B. and Schunick, W.G. (2002) *Dangerous Encounters. Avoiding Perilous Situations with Autism.* London: Jessica Kingsley Publications

Davis, C.A., Brady, M.P., Hamilton, R. and McEvoy, M.A. (1994) Effects of high-probability requests on the social interactions of young children with severe disabilities. *Journal of Applied Behavioral Analysis, 27, 619–637*

Dawson, G. and Galpert, L. (1990) Mothers' uses of imitative play for facilitating social responsiveness and toy playing in young autistic children. *Development and Psychopathology* 2, 151–162

Department of Health (2001) *Valuing People.* White Paper. London: HMSO

Frederickson, N., Warren, L. and Turner, J. (2005) Circle of Friends – An Exploration of Impact Over Time. *Educational Psychology in Practice,* 21(3), 197–217

Frith, U. (1989) *Autism:Explaining the Enigma.* Oxford: Blackwell

Gold, D. (1999) Friendship, Leisure and support: the purpose of Circles of Friends of young people. *Journal of Leisurability, 26(3)*

Grandin, T. and Scariano, M. (1986) *Emergence: Labeled Autistic.* New York: Warner Books

Gray, C. (1994) *The Social Story Book.* Texas: Future Horizons

Gray, C. (2000) *The New Social Story Book: Illustrated Edition.* Arlington, TX: Future Horizons. **www.thegraycenter.org**

Harpur, J., Lawlor, M. and Fitzgerald, M. (2006) *Succeeding with Interventions for Asperger Syndrome Adolescents.* London: Jessica Kingsley Publications

Hatton, S. (2002) A summer outing for Tom's Circle of Support. *Good Autism Practice Journal,* 3(2), 72–75

Hesmondhalgh, M. and Breakey, C. (2001) *Access and Inclusion for Children with Autistic Spectrum Disorders: Let me in.* London: Jessica Kingsley Publications

Howlin, P. (1997) *Autism: Preparing for Adulthood.* London: Routledge

Howlin, P. (2004) *Interventions for Autism: Evaluating the Evidence Base and Implementing Practical Strategies.* **www.dcpconference.co.uk/pre-conference-workshops/pre-conference-workshops_home.cfm?templatetheme=textonly**

Howlin, P. (2006) Improving Outcomes in Adult Life for People with ASD, Paper presented at Wales 2nd International Conference on ASD, Cardiff. **www.awares.org**

Howlin, P. and Goode, S. (1998) Outcome in adult life for people with autism and Asperger syndrome, in Volkmar, F. (ed.) *Autism and Pervasive Developmental Disorders.* Cambridge: University Press

Jackson, L. (2002) *Freaks, Geeks and Asperger Syndrome,* London: Jessica Kingsley Publications

Jackson, N. (2002) *Standing Down Falling Up. Asperger Syndrome from the Inside Out.* Bristol: Lucky Duck Publishing Ltd

Jamieson, J. and Jamieson, C. (2004) *Managing Asperger Syndrome at College and University. A Resource for Students, Tutors and Support Services.* London: David Fulton

Jones, J. (2000) 'Passports' to children with autism. *Good Autism Practice Journal,* 1(1), 56–65

Jordan, R.R. (1999) *Autistic Spectrum Disorders – An Introductory Handbook for Practitioners*. London: David Fulton

Kanner, L. (1943) Autistic disturbances of affective contact. *Nervous Child,* 2, 217–250

Kiker Painter, K. (2006) *Social Skills Groups for Children and Adolescents with Asperger's Syndrome*. London: Jessica Kingsley Publications

Kluth, P. (2003) *You're Gonna Love This Kid*. London: Jessica Kingsley Publications

Koegel, L.K., Koegel, R.L., Hurley, C. and Frea, W.D. (1992) Improving social skills and disruptive behavior in children with autism through self-management. *Journal of Applied Behavior Analysis,* 25, 341–353

Krantz, P.J. and McClannahan, L.E. (1993) Teaching children with autism to initiate to peers: Effects of script-fading procedure. *Journal of Applied Behavior Analysis,* 26, 121–132

LaLonde, C.E. and Chandler, M.J. (1995) False belief understanding goes to school: On the socio-emotional consequences of coming early or late to a first theory of mind. *Cognition and Emotion,* 9, 167–185

Laushey, K.M. and Heflin, J. (2000) Enhancing social skills of kindergarten children with autism through the training of multiple peers as tutors. *Journal of Autism and Developmental Disorders, 30, 183–193*

Lawson, W. (2000) *A Life Behind Glass*. London: Jessica Kingsley Publications

Lee, C. (2003) Creating a work experience programme for students with autism. *Good Autism Practice Journal,* 4(2), 37–41

Lee O'Neil, J. (1999) *Through the Eyes of Aliens*. London: Jessica Kingsley Publications

Lewis, J. (1999) Using a digital camera as an aid to developing emotional understanding in children with autism. *Good Autism Practice Journal,* September, 76–81

Lord, C. and Hopkins, J.M. (1986) The social behavior of autistic children with younger and same-age non-handicapped peers. *Journal of Autism and Developmental Disorders, 16, 249–262*

Lovaas, I. (1987) Behavioral treatment and normal intellectual and educational functioning in autistic children. *Journal of Counselling and Clinical Psychology,* 55, 3–9 (**www.lovaas.com**)

Macdonald, H., Rutter, M., Howlin, P., Rios, P., Le Couteur, A., Evered, C. and Folstein, S. (1989) Recognition and expression of emotional cues by autistic and normal adults. *Journal of Child Psychology and Psychiatry and Allied Disciplines,* 30, 865–877

Mastralengo, S. (2005) A peer-mediated buddy programme: an evaluation of process and outcomes. *Good Autism Practice Journal,* 6(1), 38–46

Mawhood, L. and Howlin, P. (1999) The outcome of a supported employment scheme for high-functioning adults with autism or Asperger syndrome. *Autism,* 3, 229–253

Mesibov, G., Shea, V. and Schopler, E. (2004) *The TEACCH Approach to autistic spectrum disorders*. New York: Plenum Press (**www.teacch.com**)

Mundschenk, N.A. and Sasso, G.M. (1995) Assessing sufficient exemplars for students with autism. *Behavioral Disorders,* 21, 62–78

Myles, Brenda Smith (2001) *Asperger Syndrome and Adolescence: Practical Solutions for School Success*. London: Jessica Kingsley Publications

Newson, E.(2000) Writing to children and young people with Asperger syndrome. *Good Autism Practice Journal,* 1(2), 17–27

Ozonoff, S. and Miller, J.N. (1995) Teaching theory of mind: A new approach to social skills training for individuals with autism. *Journal of Autism and Developmental Disorders,* 25, 415–433

Parents and Professionals Autism (PAPA) (2003) *Autistic Spectrum Disorder – A Teacher's Toolkit CD-ROM*. Belfast: Department of Education, Department of Education and Science, NI

PAPA (2005) *Connecting with Autism. Rainbow Resource Kit.* Belfast: PAPA (www. autismni.org)

Plimley, L. and Bowen, M. (2006a) *Autistic Spectrum Disorders in the Secondary School.* London: Paul Chapman Publishing, Sage

Plimley, L. and Bowen, M. (2006b) *Supporting Pupils with Autistic Spectrum Disorders – A Guide for Support Staff.* London: Sage

Plimley, L., Bowen, M. and Morgan, S.H. (2007) *Autistic Spectrum Disorders in the Early Years.* London: Sage

Potter, C. and Whittaker, C. (2001) *Enabling Communication in Children with Autism.* London: Jessica Kingsley Publications

Powell, A. (2002) *Taking Responsibility: Good Practice Guidelines for Services – Adults with Asperger Syndrome.* London: National Autistic Society

Presland, J. (1989) *Action Record for Problem Behaviour.* Kidderminster: BIMH.

Reed, P., Osborne, L. and Waddington, E.M. (2006) From lecture given by Professor Phil Reed at the 2nd International Autism Cymru conference. May 2006. Available at www.awares.org

Rinaldi, W. (1993). *The Social Use of Language Programme.* Windsor: NFER (www. wendyrinaldi.com)

Rogers, S.J. (2000) Interventions that facilitate, socialization in children with autism. *Journal of Autism and Development Disorders,* 30(5), 399–409

Sainsbury, C. (2000) *Martian in the Playground.* Bristol: Lucky Duck Publishing

Sanderson, H. (2001) It's my meeting: Finding ways to involve people with high support needs in person-centred planning. www.valuingpeople.gov.uk/documents/My-meet.pdf

Sanderson, H. (2002) *Planning with people-accessible guide.* www.helensanderson assocoates.co.uk/PDFs/What%20is%20PCP%20%20easy%20to%20read%20version.pdf

Segar, M. (1997) *Coping.* Nottingham: Early Years Centre. www.autismandcomputing. org.uk/marc2.htm

Silver, M. and Oakes, P. (2001) Evaluation of a new computer intervention to teach people with autism and Asperger syndrome to recognize and predict emotions in others. *Autism,* 5(3), 299–316

Smith, L. (2003) *Social skills training for Individuals with Autistic Spectrum Disorder: A review of the literature.* Unpublished submission to University of Birmingham, School of Education, Distance Learning Course for ASD: Children

Social Services Inspectorate (1998) *Moving into the Mainstream: The Report of a National Inspection of Services for Adults with Learning Disabilities.* London: HMSO.

Stevenson, C.L., Krantz, P.J. and McClannahan, L.E. (2000) Social interaction skills for children with autism: A script-fading procedure for non-readers. *Behavioral intervention,* 15, 1–20

Strain, P.S. and Danko, C.D. (1995) Caregivers' encouragement of positive interaction between preschoolers with autism and their siblings. *Journal of Emotional and Behavioral Disorders,* 3(1), 2–12

Szatmari, P. (2004) *A Mind Apart.* New York: Guilford Press

Tantam, D. (2000) Psychological disorder in adolescents and adults with Asperger syndrome. *Autism,* 4(1), 47–52

Waltz, M. (2005) *Metaphors of autism and autism as a metaphor.* www.inter-disciplinary.net/mso/hid/hid2/hid03s11a.htm

Wellman, J. (2005) Adolescence and sexuality presentation. Priors Court school, 7 July

Whitaker, P. (2001) *Challenging Behaviour and Autism.* London: NAS

Whitaker, P., Barratt, P., Joy, H., Potter, M. and Thomas, G. (1998) Children with autism and peer group support using circles of friends. *British Journal of Special Education,* 25(2), 60–64

White, C. (2006) *The Social Play Record*. London: Jessica Kingsley Publications

Williams, D. (1992) *Nobody, Nowhere*. New York: Time Books

Wimpory, D.C., Hobson, R.P., Williams, J.M.G. and Nash, S. (2000) Are infants with autism socially engaged? A study of recent retrospective parental reports. *Journal of Autism and Developmental Disorders,* 30(6), 525–536.

Wing, L. (1981) Asperger's syndrome. A clinical account. *Psychological Medicine*, 11, 115–130

Wing, L. (1988) The continuum of autistic characteristics, in Schopler, E. and Mesibov, G. (eds) *Diagnosis and assessment in autism*. New York: Plenum Press.

Wing, L. (1996) *The autistic spectrum*. London: Constable

Wing, L. and Gould, J. (1979) Severe impairments of social interaction and associated abnormalities in children: epidemiology and classification. *Journal of Autism and Developmental Disorders,* 9, 11–29

World Health Organisation (1993) *Mental Disorders: A Glossary and Guide to their Classification in Accordance with the 10th Revision of the International Classification of Diseases (ICD-10)*. Geneva: World Health Organisation

Zarkowska, E. and Clements, J. (1998) *Problem Behaviour and People with Severe Learning Disabilities: The S.T.A.R. Approach*. London: Nelson Thornes

Glossary

ABC	Antecedents, Behaviour, Consequences
Aetiology	The root cause of a condition or disease
AS	Asperger syndrome
ASBO	Anti-Social Behaviour Order
Autism Cymru	Wales's national charity for ASDs
CAL	Computer-assisted learning
CJS	Criminal justice system
CoF	Circle of friends
DfES	Department for Education and Skills (England)
DSM IV	*Diagnostic and Statistical Manual* (Edition 4)
GAP	*Good Autism Practice* – a journal published by the British Institute of Learning Disabilities (BILD)
ICD 10	*International Classification of Diseases*
NAS	National Autistic Society
NT	Neurotypical
PAPA	Parents and Professionals for Autism/Autism Northern Ireland, the national charity for ASDs in Northern Ireland
PCPs	Person-centred planning

PECS	Picture Exchange Communication System
PHSE	Personal, social and health education
Secondary School Forum	Developed by Autism Cymru to give teachers working with ASD in secondary schools across Wales the opportunity to meet and exchange information
SNAP Cymru	Special Needs Advisory Project in Wales
Social stories	A strategy developed by Carol Gray to teach individuals with ASD appropriate social skills
STAR	Setting, Trigger, Action, Results
SULP	Social Use of Language Programme
TEACCH	Treatment and Education of Autistic and related Communication handicapped Children
Triad of impairments	Difficulties encountered by individuals with ASD in social understanding, social communication and rigidity of thought, noted by Lorna Wing
WAG	Welsh Assembly Government

Index